A GUIDE TO COMMISSIONING HEALTH AND WELLBEING SERVICES

Amanda J. Hughes

T0342537

First published in Great Britain in 2024 by

Policy Press, an imprint of
Bristol University Press
University of Bristol
1–9 Old Park Hill
Bristol
BS2 8BB
UK
t: +44 (0)117 374 6645
e: bup-info@bristol.ac.uk

Details of international sales and distribution partners are available at
policy.bristoluniversitypress.co.uk

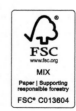

For Ava, Bailey, and Carl.

Contents

List of figures, tables, and boxes

Figures

Tables

Boxes

Acknowledgements

There are several people I would like to thank for their help as I prepared this book.

Laura Vickers-Rendall, Commissioning Editor at Policy Press, for seeing the potential and sharing my ideas for peer review.

Richard Metcalfe and Jim Manton for peer-reviewing my initial outline. Special thanks to Jim, who persuaded me there were legs to my ideas. It made a huge difference.

Katy Saunders and the team from Social Finance for sharing their work on social investment.

The palliative and end of life care team at NHS England in 2022 – the hours of work we spent on the strategy were worth it, the priorities of quality, access, and sustainability remain my key aims.

The commissioning team at One Bromley South East London Integrated Care Board – working in an integrated care system opened my eyes to commissioning challenges post COVID-19.

Carl for his patience and encouragement – I couldn't have done it without your support.

1

Introduction

About the author

I have been a commissioner in the NHS since 2009. I previously worked as an allied health professional on the frontline in neurophysiology, but I enjoyed the planning and designing side of work more than the practical hands-on aspects. I had a friend who worked in NHS commissioning, and it sounded like an interesting job and a better fit for me. A vacancy came up in a neighbouring town, but I had zero commissioning experience. However, I did my research and, luckily, the two people who interviewed me believed that enthusiasm can equal potential. The rest is history: I spent nine years in local commissioning within a clinical commissioning group and then five years in national commissioning for NHS England. I now work on an independent basis alongside many commissioning organisations. This has enabled me to learn more, spread my expertise, and be actively involved in supporting a greater number of improvements for health and social care.

Back in 2009, the clinical commissioning group I worked in was small. We had a limited team due to the small population in the area, and everybody had to cover a wide breadth of responsibilities. It was a very busy and at times hectic approach, but it gave me valuable exposure to every sector of care (acute, community, primary, voluntary, independent, and social care) and experience across multiple roles (analysis, transformation, contract negotiation, finance, quality, and so on). This meant I had the knowledge, skills, and confidence to tackle just about any commissioning problem.

In my NHS England role, I soon realised that the level of knowledge of end-to-end commissioning processes I had gained was not necessarily shared by all commissioners. The commissioners I met, especially those in larger organisations, had a specific responsibility within a particular sector of health and care. They would know their specialist area – for example, improving cancer services – inside out, but often had not had the chance to gain experience in all aspects of commissioning. For instance, they may not have in-depth knowledge of preparing a contract – they would have a separate team to complete tasks like that for them. However, this piecemeal approach to commissioning can create issues where the different commissioning functions don't have a clear understanding of how they can support each other to best effect.

As a national commissioner with NHS England, I gave commissioning advice to many people, and I was happy to do so, but in busier times I would have liked to have been able to signpost people to a good source of information on commissioning. Unfortunately, there wasn't one. The available texts tended to be heavy on academic theory or policy focused. They did little to explain the practical application of commissioning. Hence, I made a commitment to create a simple, plain language, helpful resource for people with an interest in understanding and applying commissioning for improving health and wellbeing services.

About the book

Intended audience

The aim of this book is to provide a guide to concepts and processes that are useful for people working in the commissioning of health and social care. Policy is discussed, but predominantly the book provides practical advice on how to commission well. The final chapter brings together the different aspects of the process of commissioning in a single model.

This book is valuable for:

- commissioners working within health and social care – they may be employed by the NHS at regional, national or local level, perhaps in an integrated care board, or they may be employed by local authority;
- leaders in health and social care;
- consultants or freelancers working with and for public service bodies;
- those who are studying health and social care;
- providers of health and social care who would benefit from a better understanding of the processes involved or who want to contribute more to ensure commissioning is a success;
- community leaders who would benefit from understanding how they can contribute to improving health and wellbeing through commissioning processes.

How to use the book

I am a realist and I know commissioners and people working in health and social care are busy people. Initially, I would recommend reading Chapters 2 and 3 at least, to get a good grounding of the commissioning principles. Then, if short on time, dip in and out of the chapters as needed to guide your work.

In most chapters, there are additional information boxes called 'Good to know'. These explain terms or share a little extra information on selected topics to broaden understanding. There is also a section at the end of each chapter sharing short reflections for leaders in health and social care. This may be a strategic consideration or an approach that senior leaders may find helpful to consider further. Finally, reflections are included at the end of every chapter with suggestions for success. It is easy to get caught up in the many things you have to think about and do, but I hope these reflections will help you focus on the key things to remember.

Chapter 12 summarises all the priority considerations for good commissioning and presents my simple model of outcomes-based commissioning, which I hope you will find useful as an aid to memory when planning your approach to new commissioning projects.

The context

Health and wellbeing

Commissioning has many aims, but its purpose is predominantly to establish services which improve our health and wellbeing by treating us, caring for us, or preventing our ill health and deterioration. Key here is the focus on health *and* wellbeing. This is because a focus on health alone, or absence of disease, is not enough for ensuring a 'well' population. There should be a focus on wellness, which encompasses a state of good physical, mental, emotional, and social wellbeing.

Health and wellbeing are linked. Poor experiences in one very often cause issues with the other, and there is a fine balance between the two. This connection between health and wellbeing needs has been recognised for years. In 1943, Maslow shared the hierarchy of needs, which is well recognised today. It is shared in adapted form in Figure 1.1.

Figure 1.1: Maslow's hierarchy of needs related to wellbeing

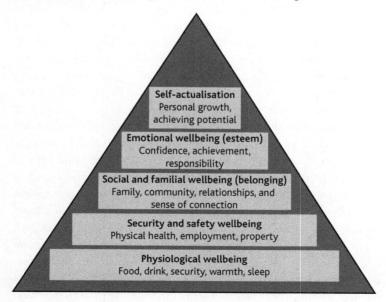

Source: Adapted from Maslow (1943) © 1943 American Psychological Association

In the hierarchy of needs, without strongly established lower tiers, we are unable to progress to the ultimate aim of self-actualisation, where we realise personal growth and achieve our potential. This highest tier is out of the reach of commissioners and providers to provide directly, but they can contribute to the lower tiers as they collaborate to meet the holistic needs of people. We will see how this can be achieved as we examine processes of commissioning throughout the book.

Therefore, commissioners need to take a holistic view of improving outcomes for people. This expands on traditional views of good physical and mental health and includes feelings of security, supportive relationships, social connectedness, economic wellbeing, and so on. Through this approach, better outcomes can be achieved and people's lives can be improved, but it can also support a sustainable health and care system that controls some of the demand by preventing, as well as responding to, ill health.

Future approaches for the NHS

In broad terms, the policy aims we see today represent a shift from traditional approaches. The commissioning vision and approaches for health and social care are centrally set out in policy and guidance by the government and NHS England – for example, in the NHS Long Term Plan (NHS England, 2019c). These documents draw on a wide interpretation of how health and care should be delivered today and in the future. They have aspirational goals, which are potentially difficult to fulfil in times of high demand and limited funding, but commissioning can shift to reflect and support these shared national aims. The following general approaches underpin much of national policy today:

- a shift from organisational silos to integrated structures – public services now aim to work collaboratively across organisational boundaries to better understand and address people's needs. The new structure of the NHS, with integrated care systems, will go some way to achieving the aim of joint working, and the Health and Care Act 2022 has removed some of the legislative barriers that previously thwarted efforts in this area (see more in Chapter 3);

- a shift from reliance on limited data to a population health management approach – the aim here is to see a move away from the focus on narrow data, such as counting people with ill health and the number of treatments provided, towards examining and understanding the wider health and wellbeing needs of a population (more in Chapter 4);
- a shift from complex funding structures to flexible, fair payment systems – in the past, a limiter for organisations working effectively together was the silo approach to funding services, with its disincentives for collaboration; Chapter 7 looks at new payment approaches in the NHS and examines how the payment model aims to facilitate joined-up working, support fairer funding, ensure greater stability, and incentivise quality and integration for improved outcomes;
- a shift from equality to equity for all – this important shift in priorities will mean there is a stronger focus on commissioning services that ensure equity of access and targeted interventions for people with different needs. Organisations will work together to promote inclusion and tackle health inequalities (see more in Chapter 9);
- a shift from a one-size-fits-all approach to personalised care – services that are personal and sensitive to individual needs, and which allow people to maintain independence, achieve better outcomes for both people and the wider care system. Personalised care approaches are now a priority for the NHS (see more in Chapter 10);
- a shift from reactive care to proactive care and prevention – prioritising the promotion of health and wellbeing and investing now to reduce future costs of ill health will improve outcomes for people and ensure sustainability of the NHS in the long term. This is a priority in public health, but commissioners elsewhere can take a similar approach as they design care services. For example, they could consider provision of patient education on self-care, prescribing initiatives to reduce the risk of deterioration among people with conditions such as high blood pressure, or initiatives

that enable communities or community groups to support groups in the population;

- a shift from care in hospitals to care closer to home – this involves building on primary and community care structures and resources to allow care and support to be wrapped around community and neighbourhood needs, providing support and care as and when it is needed. Care systems now recognise the value of care closer to home and the importance of supporting local communities for improving health and wellbeing;
- a shift from isolated planning to social impact planning – Chapter 11 looks to the priorities for health and wellbeing, now and for the future. These include the challenges of an ageing population, the impact of technological innovations, and the consequences of the global pandemic, as well as the growing need for environmental responsibility as our planet faces climate change. The impact of all these will be felt by the NHS and social care, so they will be clear priorities for strategic planning.

This book puts these shifts in thinking, and the challenges and opportunities for the future, into context for today's commissioners. It offers practical advice and guidance on how to implement change in a meaningful and effective way as part of value-based and future-facing commissioning.

The differences between health and social care

The majority of the principles of commissioning apply to both healthcare (delivered largely by the NHS) and social care (delivered by local government bodies).

Healthcare involves treatment for a specific medical condition, such as knee pain or cancer. Mental health conditions are also included. It involves some type of investigation, intervention, or care. It can also include support for self-management.

Social care involves offering people support to cope with conditions and live their lives. This includes support to go home safely after surgery and help with hygiene and eating. This support is of a practical nature and enables vulnerable persons to live as independently as possible.

Both types of care need commissioning. Typically, health and social care commissioners do their jobs separately, with only some areas of overlap. However, with the new system reforms (see Chapter 3), the relationship between them will become closer and more integrated.

2

Understanding commissioning

Aim

The aim of this chapter is to provide an overview of the commissioning process for health and social care, drawing on the well-known commissioning cycle model. The chapter covers what commissioning is, how it is beneficial, and how it works in practice.

Commissioning explained

The following is a definition of health and social care commissioning that I like – it is provided by NHS England (2024g):

> Commissioning is the continual process of planning, agreeing, and monitoring services. Commissioning is not one action but many, ranging from the health-needs assessment for a population, through the clinically based design of patient pathways, to service specification and contract negotiation or procurement, with continuous quality assessment.

The objective of commissioning for health and social care is, in simple terms, to ensure we have **the right health and social care services, for the people who need it, when and**

where they need it. And these services must be **safe, good quality, value for money, and sustainable**. That's a quite a lot to get right, and that's why commissioning can be a complex and lengthy process.

Typically, the commissioning process goes through stages of strategic planning based on local needs, designing and procuring services, and monitoring and evaluating services to make sure the aims are being achieved. These stages are described in detail later in the chapter.

The benefits of commissioning

There are many benefits of commissioning. The obvious one is that health and social care services are provided for people who need them. But if that was the only objective, then we would not need commissioners – we could just hand over all responsibility to providers and leave them to get on and deliver services. However, this would not be fully effective, due a number of reasons, explored next.

Why we need commissioners

It would be easy to question why we need commissioners, especially as national health and social care policy is promoting collaboration across multiple partners with a wider share of responsibility than we have previously been used to. However, I would argue that as partner collaboration increases, unbiased and effective commissioners are more important than ever. Good commissioners, with a focus on improving whole population health and wellbeing, have a varied role, including the responsibilities outlined next.

Carrying out widespread analysis to understand needs

Commissioners examine many sources of data and intelligence so that they can fully understand what is needed, what is happening now, and what may be coming in the future. This includes, among many other things, understanding local health needs and predicting trends for the future. This ensures that services are in place to meet current need and that there is a process of planning for services in the future. Commissioners can do this in an unbiased way for the whole population.

Coordinating collaboration

Commissioners can put into place consultation (this essentially means running ideas past people to get their views) and engagement (this means getting people actively involved in planning and designing) with multiple partners who may have an influence or impact on implementing effective services. This might be other healthcare providers, social care providers, education providers, voluntary, community and social enterprise organisations, people in the local community, or groups of people with lived experience of a health or social care need.

Why does consultation and engagement with different groups matter? We don't live in bubbles related to a single health or social care problem. And people have multiple and often complex needs – for example, a person with a long-term condition may also have depression and need help with their personal care needs at home. They need physical, mental, and social care support, and if any of these needs goes unaddressed, it can have negative impacts on the others. If commissioners don't involve other organisations to be part of the solution, then an opportunity is missed to improve health and wellbeing.

Commissioners can coordinate the different organisational voices into a whole without lending too much weight to any one sector or approach. They ensure balance. Part of that balance means listening to the people receiving the service or living within the affected community – in this way, commissioners can ensure that local voices contribute to effective change.

Collaboration is also important because introducing a service may have consequences for other services, parts of the health and social care systems, other organisations, or people close to those receiving help. Understanding intended and unintended consequences of commissioning is important to ensure that benefits are evident within the target population, that staff are supported to manage change, and that the wider system benefits.

Holding providers to account

If a provider governs itself, how can we be truly sure that it is doing a good job? And if things are going wrong, how can we know that something is being done about it?

Commissioners are part of a separate organisational body that can hold providers to account on quality, safety, and delivery within national guidelines. This governance includes the obvious concerns, such as ensuring clinical services are performing well, but it also includes oversight of issues such as value for money and protection of service users' personal data.

Holding the pursestrings

Someone needs to make sure that the finite (and dwindling) financial resources for health and social care are being used in the most effective way to help the maximum amount of people and address the greatest need. Commissioners have the unenviable job of deciding what is and isn't affordable, and ensuring that what is commissioned provides value for money. They are the organisation responsible for distributing the available money fairly and effectively among several providers to achieve the best outcomes.

How people benefit from good commissioning

So, what does good commissioning mean for people on the receiving end of health and social care services? I suggest that good commissioning can deliver a range of benefits for people, including:

- safe and effective services that may:
  - o improve quality of life for those with an illness or a condition;
  - o potentially prolong life;
  - o potentially prevent ill health or slow disease progression;
- improved experiences of health and social care through:
  - o less worry, due to trust in the provider to do a good job;
  - o reduced discomfort or pain during care or procedures;
  - o reduced waiting times;

o care closer to home;
o seamless transfers between services;
o good information about illnesses and conditions as well as the care that will be received;
• holistic approaches that:
o include personalised approaches that take the individual and their personal preferences into account;
o offer a wider view of health that includes general wellbeing and social circumstances;
o consider the wider opportunities to support people, such as community resources;
• benefits for wider society, including:
o reduced demand on health and social care services as people are treated or cared for earlier, ill health is prevented, and disease progression is slowed;
o reduced cost and increased value for money for the taxpayer due to effective financial distribution and planning;
o empowered communities that support each other with health and wellbeing needs;
o reduced waste and duplication of services;
o prevention of avoidable health inequalities, which can be identified and addressed.

How the system benefits from good commissioning

Health and social care systems benefit from good commissioning because it means the available public money is used effectively. Funding for health and social care services is provided by the Department of Health and Social Care to either integrated care boards (Chapter 3) or local government bodies. The allocation is calculated using statistical formula that weigh the needs of individual areas on factors such as size of population and demographic make-up. This aims to make the distribution fair and objective. It can be argued that the NHS and social care services have experienced years of underfunding. The NHS Confederation (2022) estimate that the funding shortfall in 2022 was somewhere between £4 billion and £9.4 billion. Recent challenges, such as COVID-19, new technology, staff pay disputes, and energy costs have hit the sector hard. Most years, with recent years being no exception, the health and social care sectors have to make efficiency savings in order to balance the books.

Commissioners have the very difficult job of delivering value for money with a very restricted budget. They aim to get the maximum impact out of limited resources, and they ensure taxpayer money is well spent. Sometimes, they must make difficult decisions regarding what they can and cannot fund. The need for skilled and experienced commissioners to ensure funding is allocated fairly and effectively is often overlooked.

The commissioning cycle

The **commissioning cycle** describes the process of commissioning. A typical cycle is presented in Figure 2.1 with three key stages; there are specific activities to be completed within each of these stages. You may come across other commissioning models that have more stages in the cycle, but for simplicity I refer to three. The nature of the process is that as one revolution of the cycle ends, the process begins again. That may sound never-ending, but it simply reflects the nature of doing and learning, applying new knowledge, and adapting to external factors. It is good practice for commissioners to stay reflective and dynamic in their approach, and to try not to see completed commissioning projects as finished, but rather as progressing.

Figure 2.1: The commissioning cycle

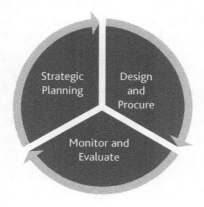

Each revolution of the cycle will vary. Sometimes a cycle can require a few years to complete, especially for a brand-new service with lots of unknown aspects. Other cycles may only require a few months, with a brief review for minor improvements. This is more likely for well-established services that have only small alterations in-year. And the process is not always linear – a catalyst for change can come at any point in the cycle, and many cycle actions might be completed simultaneously, or some stages missed completely if they are not required in a particular context. A good commissioner will be flexible to meet the needs of the project in question.

The three stages shown in Figure 2.1 are examined in more detail in Table 2.1. In the first stage – strategic planning – it is important to understand 'need'. Answering the following questions regarding need can help lay the foundation for the commissioning actions required:

- What are the health and social care needs of the population?
- What services would address those needs?
- Who, and how many people, need those services?
- When and where are those services needed?
- If introduced or altered, what impact will this service have on people, communities, or other services?

(Processes for the collection and use of data and intelligence, which support commissioners in answering these sorts of question, are outlined in Chapter 4.)

In the next stage of commissioning – design and procure – the information gathered is used to design services that meet the identified needs (more on this in Chapter 5). The aim is to implement high-quality services that are safely and skilfully staffed and affordable. Furthermore, the ideal service design allows flexibility for adapting to external factors and need for change. This may be unexpected changes in patient demand, political changes to the health and social care systems, or a global pandemic. Once local needs are understood and services have been designed services to meet and address those needs, these arrangements are captured in legal contracts that safeguard what has been designed and support effective implementation (Chapter 6).

Table 2.1: Stages in the commissioning cycle

Key activity	Details
1. Strategic Planning	
Assess local needs and priorities	This process involves accumulation of data and intelligence that shows what is happening (or not happening) locally. This shows where health and wellbeing outcomes are not optimal. The assessment also considers any local priorities (including those mentioned within system-wide strategic plans). Local strategic plans can help steer or support a project, but if the project is not a local priority, this can hinder plans to take it forward. If there is misalignment between the project and local priorities, it is important to be aware of this. (Assessment of needs is examined more closely in Chapter 4.)
Identify national priorities	In addition to local priorities, there will be national priorities that may influence the commissioning process. It's important to be aware of these, because there may be mandatory obligations on the commissioner to do something locally, or there may be opportunities for support (funding, networks, or guidance) if a proposed project is backed up by national programmes. National priorities are usually defined within the NHS operational planning guidance. This is published every year to share national priorities with those planning and delivering care for the coming year.
Map existing provision and resources	Before identified needs can be addressed, it is necessary to understand what services or provisions are already in place. What are the gaps? What is working well or not well? It may be there is already provision or good practice in place that the commissioner was unaware of. This may mean there is no need to do anything new. Or it may be that alteration to existing services is an effective option.
Confirm needs and priorities with partners and service users	There will often be things that data can't show. This might be an unidentified need or a barrier that limits access to services. This is why talking to a range of people who have or will be – or should be – using the services is important. (This is examined as part of co-production in Chapter 5.)
2. Design and Procure	
Design services	Now that the local needs and gaps are understood, the commissioner can start to design how these will be addressed. (This process is covered in Chapter 5.) Essentially, they will be specifying what the service will do, to whom, when, and where. Ideally this will be presented in a service specification.
Ensure supply	Once the design is finalised, either the change is delivered by an existing provider (incumbent) or a new provider is identified to deliver it. There are a few routes to achieve this. If the change is significant (very different from current provision and/or costs a lot of money), the commissioner is bound by procurement rules and may need to offer the service to all interested parties via procurement routes. If the change is not significant, or there is reasonably only one provider that can provide this service, the commissioner can ask an existing provider to implement it.

Table 2.1: Stages in the commissioning cycle (continued)

Key activity	Details
Contract for assurance	For both new and existing providers, the NHS standard contract is used to enact the change. This ensures there is clear and transparent agreement on what the service provision includes, how it will be paid for, and what the quality and information standards are. It provides legal protection for the provider and the commissioner. (Contracts are discussed in Chapter 6.)
Implement delivery	The implementation process requires a very clear service design, which is usually shared in a service specification, and a detailed implementation plan. Implementation plans usually include any prerequisites for delivery, such as recruitment of staff, training, and equipment. Then, depending on scale, the change is rolled out with clear milestones charting progress. Referrers and patients need to be informed about the changes. Supporting infrastructure, such as shared care records or administration processes, is carefully planned and introduced.

3. Monitor and Evaluate	
Monitor delivery performance	During design of the service, the commissioner sets out how it is to be monitored and evaluated. There are three main aspects to evaluating a service: a) Is the provider doing the job they have been asked to do in a way that is safe and gives value for money? b) Do the expected outcomes match the expectations for people's needs – for example, are patients having a good experience and achieving good clinical outcomes? c) Can anything be improved? Chapter 8 looks at evaluation in detail, but for now the main point is that this part of the cycle is essential – there cannot be learning and growth without it.
Feed learning into stage 1, with the aim of improving, reshaping, or decommissioning the service	Here, we are back at the beginning of the cycle but with the advantage of having the changes in place, process learning, and improved data and intelligence following evaluation. The commissioner may need to make some minor tweaks to improve the service, or they may need to make big changes to achieve the impact they sought. In some extreme cases, they may have to decommission (withdraw permission and funding for the service; see more in Chapter 6) and start from scratch. This is rare, but if it does happen, there will be lots of learning to take away. Where the change has been a success, the commissioner should share the learning with others, celebrate the success, and look to scale up where possible.

Funding arrangements ensure the service is financially sustainable and can act as a lever to incentivise high-quality provision (Chapter 7).

The next stage – monitoring and evaluation – is carried out to assure that the aims have been achieved (Chapter 8). The evaluation process provides further information and intelligence, feeding into a continuous cycle of activities.

Length of the commissioning cycle

All commissioning projects and programmes are different, and the length of the commissioning cycle varies accordingly. A small or very urgent change can be implemented in a month or two, while a large-scale change typically takes place over several years.

Procurement processes, where needed, can take considerable time – up to and over a year in some cases – but again this depends on scale. Due to all the legal steps required, the minimum period for procurement is usually three months (for more detail, see Chapter 6).

Typical commissioning calendar

Usually, the commissioning cycle is yearly and coincides with the contracting timetable for each financial year (April to March). The year is divided into three-month periods: quarters one, two, three, and four. Quarter one starts in April.

In recent years, there has been a shift to two-year or longer contract deals, and in these cases the commissioning cycle coincides with this timeframe. This longer period aims to create stability for the provider and reduce the administration burden for all. This can be a helpful approach, and many contract schedules can be agreed for a two-year plus period. However, some elements will likely need fresh negotiation at the end of the first 12 months, and the commissioning cycle evaluation will highlight where improvements can be made. Other aspects of a contract that are likely to need a revisit every year include indicative activity plans and the funding envelope to match these activity levels. There will also be a need to enact any new national guidance into the contract. So multi-year contracts are useful in principle, but don't remove the need for annual review and refresh.

A summary of the typical timetable for commissioning and contracting activities is provided in Table 2.2, but remember that

Table 2.2: The commissioning and contracting yearly timetable

Quarter	Months	Activity
Quarter one	April, May, June	Contracts are signed. All parties settle into the new arrangements – collaboration is required to sort out teething problems. Monthly contract monitoring meetings are established.
Quarter two	July, August, September	Data reporting is usually well established by now, as providers will have trained staff on data collection processes and will have implemented any new systems and requirements. Quarter one data should start to flow to commissioners.
Quarter three	October, November, December	Planning for the next year begins. Contract intentions from commissioners and providers are shared – these are summaries of what they wish to negotiate for the next year. The negotiation period for local priorities usually begins now. The NHS operational planning and contracting guidance, which sets out national priorities, is due in December.
Quarter four	January, February, March	This is a very busy time for completing contracting schedules and agreeing financial budgets. Contracts should be signed before 31 March, but NHS England provides timescales yearly.

the stages may not be linear – for example, there may be contract amendments that enact changes mid-year or before a new contract is signed (more on this in Chapter 6).

REFLECTIONS FOR LEADERS

Strategic value of the commissioning cycle

The commissioning cycle is useful for leaders in health and social care as the overall process informs strategy and, conversely, strategy informs the focus of a commissioning cycle. To support this process of information exchange, ensure a framework is in place for communicating identified priorities throughout the commissioning team, including senior decision makers.

Strategy can and should be steered by national priorities and policy, but local intelligence provides the context, justification for change, and evidence and gives meaning to what you are aiming to do. The importance of local intelligence, and gathering of it, is sometimes overlooked, so build in processes for sharing the learning from:

- population health analyses;

- design processes;

- engagement with people;

- service evaluations.

Suggestions for success

Embrace the cyclical process of commissioning. Don't be disheartened by the fact that commissioned projects are never truly finished. Keep in mind that, like many things in life, this is an evolving process and there is always room for improvement.

Don't let traditional commissioning timetables stand in the way of starting to identify and design improvements, because, first, you can underestimate how long the process from issue to implementation takes and, second, a change can be enacted at any time with the agreement of providers and the right contractual processes. Why wait if it will bring benefits?

3

England's health commissioning model

Aim

This chapter examines the model of commissioning used currently in England. It provides a detailed discussion of the integrated care system established legally in 2022 and all the partner organisations that are required to collaborate to make this approach effective. It also briefly outlines commissioning models in the other countries of the UK, and some international examples, to see how they compare with the model in England.

The commissioning model in England

In the early 1990s, health reforms in England moved to separate the purchasing of services from their delivery. This created an 'internal market', meaning health and care providers operate like a business. The intention was to create efficiencies via a more competitive market that has a clear 'purchaser–provider' arrangement. Simply put, commissioners purchase services from the health and care providers. This arm's-length approach was strengthened in 2012 with the finalisation of the Transforming Community Services programme and the implementation of the Health and Social Care Act 2012. Prior to this, the only providers not in a purchaser–provider arrangement were community services, which were entwined with the commissioning bodies, then called primary care trusts. The Transforming Community Services programme sought to separate the community services element from primary care trusts into distinct providers, severing the organisational link. Clinical commissioning groups were then formed, replacing primary care trusts.

The rhetoric for the internal market reforms in the 1990s and 2012 was about improving quality with new arrangements that would be more efficient, responsive, and innovative. The *BMJ* (Moberly, 2018) reported the British Medical Association (BMA) argument that these reforms were more to do with saving money via structural change and greater competition. The BMA made a call to repeal the changes made in 2012, at their annual representative meeting. Segall (2018), in line with the earlier BMA position, argues that this move towards separation was not effective. He notes that the internal market creates higher regulatory and transaction costs, greater fragmentation between services, and more bureaucracy, and that it invites opportunities for privatisation.

My opinion has been formed during my employment in both a primary care trust and a clinical commissioning group. I suggest that there have been good and bad outcomes from the internal market, and as ever we learn through the journey. In my experience, the separation of purchaser and provider has led to a clearer process for holding providers to account for quality and delivery, though it is perhaps not an easier process, due to the relationship divides that have been created. There is sometimes lack of transparency, due to mistrust between parties. Privatisation and competition opportunities have opened the door in some health and care areas to more innovative approaches, greater choice for patients, and the alleviation of stress in some high-demand sectors of health and care. But, conversely, the process for managing competition takes much longer and hence costs more, and it has created organisational barriers between providers where care should be seamless. Finally, I will add that although providers, whether NHS or private, can potentially have more freedom to operate efficiently within the internal market model, there are risks of them being driven by the wrong incentives, with choices being made primarily for financial gain, opportunities for cost efficiencies at scale being lost due to fragmentation, and patients being cherry-picked or held onto too long due to financial reasons.

The Health and Care Act 2022 introduced legislation to transform the NHS yet again. This time the aim is to make the system less bureaucratic and more integrated. The Act seems to be reversing some of the structural changes of the 1990s and 2012 with a move to greater collaboration between commissioners and providers, and loosening of some of the competition and tendering rules. The purchaser–provider split still operates, but the lines are more blurred. In my opinion this is a positive step. The new model aims to make it easier for organisations to deliver joined-up care for people who often have many complex health, wellbeing, and care needs; it aims to ease some of the financial juggling by ensuring financial arrangements are more transparent and for the greater good of the system; and it aims to support the goals of the NHS, such as reducing unwarranted inequalities and improving personalised care approaches, through joint working. Inevitably, there are challenges with any large-scale reform, and I cover these later in the chapter.

In addition to the changes for the NHS, the new Act introduces social care reforms, such as the 'cap-and-floor model' (Department of Health and Social Care, 2022a) for personal social care costs. This aims to reduce some of the uncertainty people face with social care costs. A higher 'cap' – that is, the maximum value anyone will have to pay towards their personal care costs in their lifetime – was brought in. The 'floor' is the point at which people must contribute to these costs, and this rises in value increments up to 100 per cent for those with greater assets. People with a low value of assets will never have to contribute to their personal care costs. The fairness of these changes is debatable, as those with financial assets well in excess of the 100 per cent floor will be significantly less affected than someone who only just reaches the threshold. Torsten Bell (2021), of the Resolution Foundation think tank, tweeted after the government plans were first unveiled: 'Here's a simple way to think about the problem … : if you own a £1m house in the home counties, over 90% of your assets are protected. If you've got a terraced house in Hartlepool (worth £70k) you can lose almost everything.' I agree this aspect is unfair, but that said, I believe that, though the thresholds create unfair consequences for some, the general direction of reform is right - it seeks to support more people with care costs and address the uncertainty of what they have to pay.

The structure of commissioning for health in England

There are several tiers of commissioning within the NHS. Table 3.1 sets out the key tiers and the associated responsibilities. Be mindful, though, that the NHS doesn't stand still for long – there are changes in structures and systems every ten years or so.

Table 3.1: Commissioning tiers

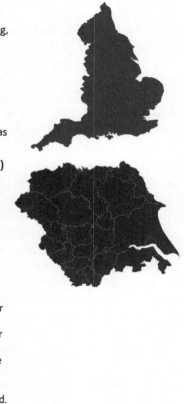

National (NHS England)
NHS England is the organisation with interests in ensuring good commissioning, and subsequently good care and outcomes, across England. They provide the policy position and national strategy which sets the focus for all the commissioning bodies in the system. They play a helpful role in designing and supporting transformation across the country, specifically supporting regions as they develop system transformation.

Regional (NHS England regional teams)
There are seven NHS regions in England. Each has an NHS England regional team that supports development and holds integrated care systems to account in quarterly meetings. These regional teams feed information to the central NHS England teams to ensure policy and strategy is informed by system-level commissioning.
Regional teams support practical commissioning for a regional footprint. For example, a regional team might support arrangements for a highly specialist cancer service that all systems in the region pay towards. When care is commissioned once across a region, rather than several times for each system, costs can be shared and higher standards of quality can be achieved. These range from 5.7m to over 14m each.

Table 3.1: Commissioning tiers (continued)

Subregions (integrated care systems)
As of 2022, integrated care systems are the key commissioning bodies for health. They bring together local authorities and other partners in a coordinated effort to create conditions for joined-up health and social care commissioning. The aim is improved outcomes for their populations, specifically in relation to health and wellbeing. This approach, with a wide geographical area covered by one integrated care system, is deemed beneficial for reducing unwarranted variation in care and outcomes, as best practice is implemented across the system.

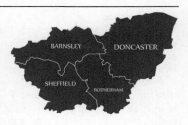

Integrated care systems have NHS-led **integrated care boards**, which are responsible for the governance and accountability arrangements for health services across the system. These manage performance and collective finance arrangements. **Integrated care partnerships** are the vehicles for joining together care bodies, with the NHS and local authorities working together with other interested parties to improve the health and wellbeing of people at subregion level.
Per subregion, commissioning covers services for 500,000 to three million people.

Place
Places include health and wellbeing boards and place-based partnerships. These are often geographically aligned with the integrated care board and local authority. Historically, these footprints were the domain of the former clinical commissioning groups working alongside local government partners.
Commissioning at this level has oversight of local services that are specific to the place. It may involve integrating services across hospital, council and primary care teams for anticipatory care or hospital discharge.
Per place, commissioning covers services for approximately 250,000 to 500,000 people.

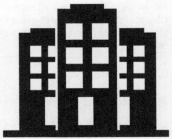

(continued)

Table 3.1: Commissioning tiers (continued)

Neighbourhood
Smaller still are 'neighbourhoods' which are important tiers of the system but are less well defined – here, primary care works alongside multidisciplinary community health teams or social care in the form of primary care networks. The local VCSE sector and community-based initiatives are active here and contribute to a close-knit approach to keeping people well and supported.
Neighbourhoods have a proactive role in population health and prevention, and they draw on resources from the community and VCSE sector.

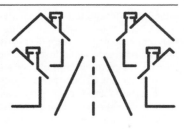

Per neighbourhood, commissioning covers services for approximately 30,000 to 50,000 people.

Individuals
Commissioning usually covers services for (mostly large) groups of people, but there are some exceptions.
Personalised care approaches consider what matters to each person, and subsequently care is designed specifically for the individual.
Another example of individual care is requests for treatment that is not routinely funded. Funding can be granted for specialist treatment if an individual's clinical circumstance is very unique. These are known as 'individual funding requests'.

Integrated care systems

At the time of writing this book, we are settling into a new arrangement of integrated care systems. These are partnerships that bring together NHS organisations, local authorities, and others to take a shared responsibility for planning services, improving health, and reducing inequalities across a particular geographical area. The four key NHS England policy aims for integrated care systems are (NHS England, 2023a):

- improving outcomes in population health and health care;
- tackling inequalities in outcomes, experience, and access;
- enhancing productivity and value for money;
- helping the NHS to support broader social and economic development.

These aims will be familiar to health and social care commissioners, with the addition of the wider consideration of what local communities need to flourish.

In 2023, there were 42 integrated care systems across England, each covering populations in the region of 500,000 to three million people. Figure 3.1 shows the regional footprints, each with an integrated care system.

The structure of the integrated care system looks something like the arrangement in Figure 3.2. At system level there is the dual structure of integrated care board and integrated care partnership, both of which are influenced by and work alongside the other bodies within the system. They work closely with health and wellbeing boards, primary care networks, and provider collaboratives in their area. This structure aims to allow these varied organisations, with their separate statutory duties and governance structures, to find ways of working together effectively.

The various components of an integrated care system are described next.

Integrated care boards

Integrated care boards are the statutory bodies responsible for planning and funding most NHS services in the areas covered by integrated care systems. They have legal responsibilities in this regard and are accountable to NHS England. National policy dictates that the membership of an integrated care board includes a chair, a chief executive officer, and at least three other members from local NHS trusts, general practice, and local authorities. In addition, at least one member must have knowledge and expertise in mental health services. The board can also include leaders from the private sector. The membership should ensure that no single voice is be able to influence decision making unduly. This diversity of membership, with both commissioners and providers, aims to support partnership working.

Figure 3.1: NHS regional footprints

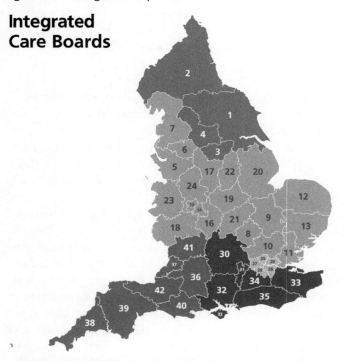

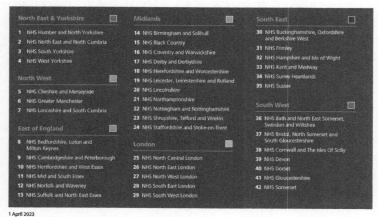

Source: NHS England (2023a) Open Government Licence v3.0

Figure 3.2: Structure of an integrated care system

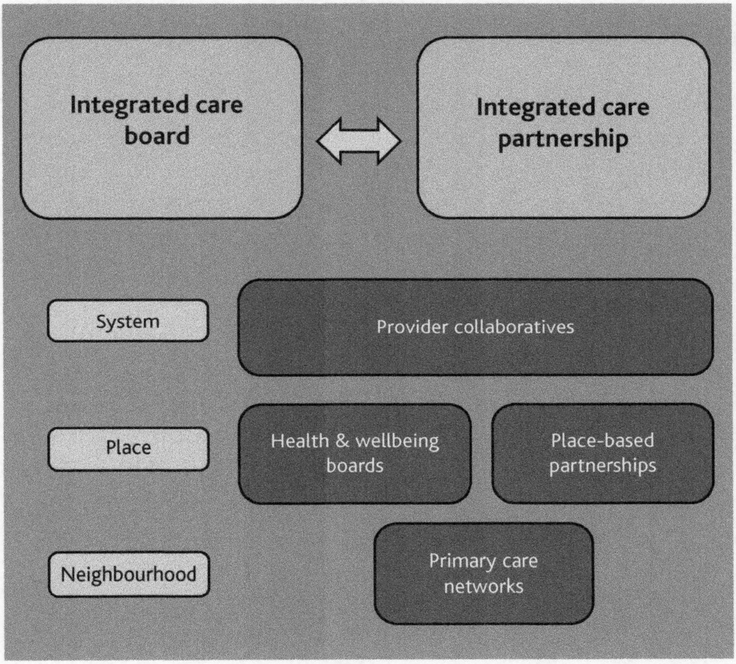

Each board must prepare a five-year plan setting out how it will meet the health needs of its population. This plan must be informed by the health and wellbeing strategies published by health and wellbeing boards in their area, and it must have regard for the recommendations and priorities highlighted by the integrated care partnership.

Integrated care partnerships

Integrated care partnerships are statutory committees that bring together a broad set of partners that are locally defined but predominantly include the local authorities in the area. Other partners might be providers in the NHS, public health, housing, education, the justice system, and the voluntary, community and social enterprise (VCSE) sector, and Healthwatch (an independent statutory body that speaks on behalf of people in an area in relation to health and social care). Collectively, the partners aim to develop a health and care strategy for the area. The strategy builds on joint strategic needs assessments provided by health and wellbeing strategies and health and wellbeing boards.

Integrated care partnerships can determine their own membership and their own ways of working. However, they must have at least one member from the integrated care board and one member from each local authority in the area.

Provider collaboratives

The requirement for provider collaboratives, which operate at system level, is set out in the integrated care system design framework (NHS England and NHS Improvement, 2021). These consist of groups of providers with two or more NHS trusts or foundation trusts. The providers work together to plan, deliver, and transform their services. This partnership work aims to:

- save money across a patch by working on a larger scale than they have previously – they can share back office functions, reduce duplication, and share access to equipment or staff resources;
- reduce unwarranted variation, make improvements, and deliver the best care for patients and communities – this can be achieved in part by working closely with and supporting the work of clinical networks or alliances;
- share learning and good practice;
- enable a smoother journey for patients as they move between services provided by different organisations. For the patient, this can potentially mean fewer delays, having to tell their story only once, and having accurate information about what comes next for them.

Provider collaboratives are required to agree specific objectives with the integrated care system, and they contribute to the delivery of that system's strategic priorities. How this is achieved is agreed locally, within each collaborative.

The VCSE alliance model is an example of a provider collaborative. This is examined more closely in Chapter 5.

Health and wellbeing boards

Health and wellbeing boards were established in 2013 with the aim of joining up work at a place level. The Health and Care Act 2022 introduced these boards as part of the architecture of the new integrated care system. They play an important role in facilitating joint working and setting strategic direction.

Health and wellbeing boards are statutory committees of the local authority and include representation from professional, clinical, political, and community leaders. This composition is similar to that of integrated care partnerships, but the boards are smaller in scale and represent specific places within local authorities – an integrated care partnership can encompass several health and wellbeing boards.

The boards develop the joint strategic needs assessments for the area. These are assessments of the current and future health and social care needs of a community, providing an evidence base that informs the local health and wellbeing board joint local health and wellbeing strategy, which is the vision and actions agreed by the board to improve the health and wellbeing of the community. The integrated care boards must have regard for the joint strategic needs assessments and the joint local health and wellbeing strategy, as they have a bearing on their local plans and are relevant for whole-system planning and actions.

Place-based partnerships

Place-based partnerships, focused on specific locations within the integrated care system area, can include a variety of collaborations. They usually include local authority and other local partners, such as place-based providers or VCSE organisations. These partnerships are responsible for arranging and delivering local health and care services. They serve as the foundations for the statutory system-level structures, as they can build on existing knowledge, relationships, and arrangements.

The footprint of place-based partnerships and their governance arrangements and functions are agreed at local level. These partnerships work together to achieve:

- local strategy and planning – as these place-based bodies know and understand their population well they can agree a shared vision which targets key priorities identified in population health analysis in a locally effective way;
- service planning and operational collaboration;
- identification of community assets that can be shared;
- increased community resilience and independence;
- better health and wellbeing, and prevention of ill health.

Primary care networks

Primary care networks are arrangements for joint working between a primary care provider, or providers, and additional services, such as community, mental health, pharmacy, social care, and VCSE sector services. They are general practice led. Primary care networks are a policy priority in the NHS Long Term Plan (NHS England, 2019c), and the five-year general practitioner (GP) contract introduced in 2019 (NHS England, 2019a) provides a framework to support development of these networks. The intention of policy on the networks is to promote working together to care for people proactively rather than reactively. This is especially important for people under the care of their GP for multiple long-term conditions, such as diabetes or heart disease. Supporting and caring for people holistically, rather than focusing on a condition, is also supported by the Fuller Report (Fuller, 2022; see this chapter's 'reflections for leaders').

The primary care networks, as set out in the five-year framework, aim to be proactive, coordinated, and personalised. They serve people and communities at neighbourhood level. These communities tend to be in the region of 30,000 to 50,000 people, but the size of a network can vary significantly, depending on various factors. Ideally, they need to be large enough to achieve economies of scale but small enough to tailor to local needs and allow for personalised approaches.

The challenges for integrated care systems

Although most would agree the aims of the integrated care systems are appropriate and will bring many benefits, there are some challenges that those within the (still new) structure face.

First, the integrated care systems across England are in different stages of development. Some have been operating in shadow form (non-statutory but operating like an integrated care system) from as early as 2017. Eight areas led the 'first wave' to develop system-wide collaboration, despite there not being any formal guidance in place. The aim was to share learning and understanding of the journey from clinical commissioning groups to the integrated care system model. Many other commissioning bodies established integrated care systems in 2023. It is fair to say that the full function of these later groups is not fully established in many areas. Therefore, there will be some inconsistency across integrated care systems in their preparedness to enact their statutory responsibilities well. Due to the different maturity levels, results will probably vary from area to area in the next few years.

Second, although working together means sharing the design and implementation of good care, inevitably it also means sharing the risk. This risk-sharing will add to the complexity of the relationships and the governance requirements. Additionally, different partners will have different attitudes to risk. A large acute trust that is financially struggling may welcome a partnership approach to ease their burden, but a smaller provider may have understandable concerns about financial, operational, and clinical implications.

Third, the concept of integrated care is laudable, but there needs to be a solid infrastructure in place to enable this. It requires, among many things, sharing of patient records on compatible IT systems, effective processes for timely transfers of care, good understanding of what has come before and what comes next, joint premises, and professionals who can work across more than one organisation. This infrastructure will take time and money to implement, notwithstanding the management of culture change for staff and people.

The fourth challenge of note is the political and organisational arrangements which the partners operate in. An example of this is the means-testing of some social care provision. The operating model for this provision of care, the national and local politics, the access and entry points, and many other factors will be different from health provision. If there is appetite to integrate health and social care to a greater degree, then aspects like this will take time for all the parties to understand and then successfully address.

Good to know: Specialised commissioning

Specialised commissioning is used for the planning and funding of highly specialist services for people who have rare or complex conditions. Examples include treatment for rare cancers, diagnosis of genetic disorders, and provision of specialist medical investigations. Because of how specialised these are, treatments and diagnostics are only available in a small number of locations. This is because of the highly skilled professionals, resources, and equipment they require, the very small number of people needing it, and the expense of providing it. Because of these limitations, these services are usually commissioned regionally or nationally. Currently, the need for specialised services is rising because of the ageing population and increasing advancement in medical research and technology.

At the time of writing, specialised commissioning is undergoing changes in how it is delivered and by whom. There is a recognition that although there are difficulties in commissioning these services at a system level, they still need to be joined up with other local care for the best possible outcomes. NHS England are committed to integrating the specialist commissioning arrangements within integrated care systems and have shared a roadmap for achieving this (see NHS England and NHS Improvement, 2022b). The handover of commissioning responsibilities will be phased and proportionate. Delegation of these duties began in 2023.

(See more on specialised services at: www.england.nhs.uk/commission ing/spec-services/.)

Stakeholders in commissioning

The commissioner

At present, there are no minimum requirements or standardised training for being a commissioner. Generally, people enter this area with some health project or business management experience or a public policy background, or they may have been working on the frontline in health and social care. There are no minimum qualifications, but as you progress there is expectation of a postgraduate qualification or equivalent. This means the door is wide open for this role, which is complex, requires specific skills, and is often demanding. There are positives to this in that someone with the right aptitude and general skills will not have barriers to accessing a career in commissioning, but there are risks in that it may be possible to become a commissioner without having a basic understanding of the theory and principles underpinning the responsibilities.

The job can require:

- people and collaboration skills;
- knowledge of how to use data and intelligence;
- strategic thinking;
- understanding of and ability to work within a political context;
- design and innovation skills;
- ability to manage finance and procurement;
- evaluation and research skills;
- values and behaviours conducive to improving experiences for patients and staff;
- ability and resilience to manage complex projects.

Once in a commissioning role, there are options available for development, including:

- The NHS Confederation, a membership organisation that supports and speaks for all healthcare bodies, offers a network for people working in integrated care systems (see NHS Confederation, 2024). This independent network provides a forum for collaboration and exchange of ideas and support.
- There are academic courses which offer health or social sciences training and development, including postgraduate courses for health and social care leadership.
- You can access academic modules from other sources, such the commissioning and personalised care courses delivered by the Healthcare Financial Management Association.
- The government-led Commissioning Academy (Cabinet Office, 2016) is available for public sector commissioners. This invites

commissioners from health and local government to attend courses exploring key commissioning topics. This offer reflects that there is some forward thinking within government in terms of upskilling and preparing commissioners for the future.

Clinical commissioners

Clinical commissioners have a clinical background. They may come from any discipline, but people in these roles are often doctors or nurses. These commissioners maintain their professional registration and usually continue working on a clinical basis part of the time. Clinical commissioners have increased in number since the introduction of the premise of clinical commissioning and clinical commissioning groups in 2012, but there has been a step away from this approach with the Health and Care Act 2022.

Clinical commissioners can take any commissioning role, but are usually aligned with a specific programme that matches their clinical speciality or are employed on a strategic planning basis. Clinical commissioners can be a benefit to a commissioning team as they can provide expert insight into how things operate on the ground and what will and won't work. Plus, they can be excellent voices of persuasion when it comes to other professionals who may be resistant to change or struggle to see the potential benefits for their them or their patients of the change.

Other partners in commissioning

The key partners in commissioning will vary according to the aims and plans. However, commissioners will nearly always have providers as priority partners. This may include current (incumbent) providers, providers of aligned services, or potential new providers. Providers can be from many different types of service and organisation, the most common being:

- acute services;
- community services;
- mental health services;
- primary care, including dentistry and eye care;
- social care;

- public health, including health visitors, school nurses, sexual health workers, and substance misuse workers;
- VCSE organisations;
- hospices;
- nursing homes and residential homes;
- ambulance and patient transport;
- pharmacy.

Commissioners may also have partners with links or interdependencies to a service. These can be numerous and include some of those mentioned earlier plus:

- national charities;
- schools, academies;
- local employers;
- local authority departments, such as housing or children's services;
- justice services;
- carer organisations;
- IT or data services;
- neighbouring commissioning areas (at neighbourhood, place, or integrated care system level);
- regional commissioning teams;
- national NHS England programme teams;
- suppliers of material goods.

Then, internally, the commissioning team will likely benefit from people with expertise in:

- commissioning;
- contracting;
- finance;
- data and intelligence;
- quality;
- safeguarding;
- IT;
- communications and engagement.

By now, the room is filling up! It may be that people need to be brought in and out at specific points in the commissioning cycle. Or a tiered approach might help, with a small team focusing on the day-to-day activity and a wider consultation group with opportunity to influence and add to the detail. Stakeholder analysis can assist with decisions about who needs to be involved, in what way, and at what stage.

Good to know: Public health

Public health in England has undergone some changes over the last ten years. In 2013, it was separated from the NHS and was moved to local authority governance. This change was controversial in that it created a split between care and prevention services. Today, as a result of the Health and Care Act 2022, public health duties are the responsibility of two new organisations: the Office for Health Improvement and Disparities and the UK Health Security Agency. Both organisations sit within the Department of Health and Social Care. There is commitment nationally to align the public health contribution more closely with that of the NHS and the wider care system. To that end, NHS England is taking on some of the public health duties, and the split of public health duties is as follows:

- The UK Health Security Agency is responsible for health promotion functions (see www.gov.uk/government/organisations/uk-health-secur ity-agency).
- The Office for Health Improvement and Disparities is responsible for health improvement and functions relating to the wider determinants of health and health inequalities (see www.gov.uk/government/organi sations/office-for-health-improvement-and-disparities).
- NHS England is responsible for public health delivered by health care services, including vaccination, immunisation, and screening (see (www. england.nhs.uk/commissioning/pub-hlth-res/).

The new integrated care systems are responsible for ensuring that the system includes public health partners and that it acts on public health priorities.

Stakeholder analysis

Stakeholder analysis is a good idea for larger service design or transformation programmes. This helps identify key individuals who have impact, interest, and influence. By identifying the right people at an early stage, not only can the benefits of their expertise and influence be reaped sooner, but also conflict and delays due to not involving key people may be avoided.

There are many guides to stakeholder analysis available, but the main steps are described next.

In Step 1, make a list of all the people and groups that could be affected by the area of change being examined. The list will vary from project to project, but here are some categories to ensure all the relevant people are considered:

- commissioners – the local authority or health commissioners, plus neighbouring commissioning bodies and regional commissioning support teams;
- service users – those who will be using the service;
- providers – incumbent providers plus any providers with relevant links to the service delivery and/or pathway;
- other contributors to the service – those who provide essential aspects of the service, such as ambulance or pharmacy;
- commentators – those whose opinions of the organisation are heard by service users and others; these might be local Members of Parliament or representatives of charitable bodies or of Healthwatch;
- third party consumers – those who are connected to the service users: for example, patient families;
- champions – those who believe in and will actively promote the project;
- competitors – those working in the same area who offer similar or alternative services.

Note that there will be a crossover, with people and groups fitting into more than one category.

In Step 2, prioritise the stakeholders in terms of power, influence, and the extent to which they are likely to have an impact. This can then guide the approach for each. The matrix in Table 3.2 provides a guide on how to prioritise different stakeholder groups. Where there are many different stakeholders, a column for moderate impact could be added with further forms of action.

Table 3.2: Stakeholder analysis

	Low impact	High impact
High power	**Satisfy** Ensure that these groups are well informed and that you are in contact regularly.	**Manage and involve** These groups need to be fully engaged with the process. They should be actively involved or at least fully consulted and communicated with.
Low power	**Monitor** If time and resources are limited, these groups can receive minimal updates or no updates.	**Inform and empower** These groups may need some organising – for example, active consultation with patients. Steps to increase their influence will be beneficial.

In Step 3, gain an understanding of the key stakeholders to guide the engagement approach and improve the chances of success. These prompts can be useful:

- What is their readiness for change? Classifying people in terms of their being 'in favour', 'neutral', or 'opposed' to an approach can show where there's a need for persuasion and influence.
- What emotional interest do they have?
- What financial interest do they have?
- What other motivations do they have?
- What information do they want, and how do they want to receive it?
- What is their current opinion of the area in question? Is this accurate?
- Who influences them? Do those people need to be key stakeholders too?
- What might convince them if they are opposed to an aspect of the approach?
- How can you manage their opposition, if not altered by initial attempts to convince them?
- Who will be influenced by their opinions? Do they need to be key stakeholders too?

In Step 4, build effective relationships and gain trust. Where there is trust, people work together more easily. It can build confidence, minimise uncertainty, and speed up the decision-making process. There are a range of behaviours that can help develop relationships and trust.

- Be clear, honest, and transparent.
- Be open to learning, and consider new ideas and opinions.
- Build trust by being straightforward, admitting mistakes, and keeping promises.
- Have empathy with others and show vulnerability (when appropriate).
- Let go of grievances and historical issues.
- Be consistent in thought and action.
- Think about how you can help stakeholders and not just your project.

The processes of stakeholder analysis and the building of relationships may take time, but the benefits are real and can have a great impact on success.

Involving the community

To ensure services truly meet people's needs, it is important to talk and listen to the people who have or will be – or should be – using the services in question. This is now routinely recognised as good practice.

Two key groups of people that must be engaged with – meaning proactively seek to understand their needs, invite them to contribute to designing the solution, and allow them to evaluate the change in ways that matter to them – are people in the community and people with lived experience pertinent to the area of service improvement.

People in the community

People who live or work in a community have an insight into local needs, They may also have an understanding of barriers to service delivery, such as cultural differences and access issues (for example lack of buses, need for interpreters), opportunities for service delivery, perhaps making use of existing community assets and support, and many other local factors that could affect efforts for improvement in health and wellbeing. As well as residents and those employed in the area, it would be useful to engage with communities of religious faith that meet locally and parents of children attending local schools.

People with lived experience

People who have used or are using services similar to the one being planned, and those who have lived or are living with a particular condition being targeted should also be engaged with. They have 'lived' experienced and understand what works and what doesn't work in different contexts. These people are like gold dust when it comes to both understanding what is needed and shaping effective solutions for the future.

There are many ways of involving people with lived experience in commissioning. This should be done in a meaningful way, taking the level of change into account. For example, when reviewing existing services which evaluate well on outcomes, a survey as the commissioning cycle restarts might suffice. For a large-scale change, with intentions for a brand-new service, an engagement event might be appropriate, or people with lived experience might be invited to attend working groups as the service design is in process.

In some instances, the people it is important to engage with will require advocates. This may be an adult acting on behalf of their children, a spokesperson for a community whose first language is not English, or a loved one of someone receiving end of life care. (I outline how to work effectively with people in the community and how to co-produce services in Chapter 5.)

Good to know: Healthwatch

Healthwatch, an independent body that is funded and accountable to local authorities, speak on behalf of local people in relation to health and social care matters. They act as an advocate for people who use any NHS health or social care service. Their mission is to improve people's experiences and make care better.

Their aims include:

- supporting people to speak about bad outcomes or experiences – and helping them access the advice they need;
- supporting decision makers (commissioners and partners) to both act on the feedback people share and involve communities in decisions that affect them;
- building a strong Healthwatch movement.

There are local Healthwatch bodies across England. These are led by the Healthwatch England Committee, which is a statutory committee of the Care Quality Commission (CQC). They are therefore ideally placed to escalate any concerns to the CQC, and they can advise national organisations, such as the government and NHS England, about the quality of services. (See more at the Healthwatch website: www.healthwatch.co.uk/)

Comparing commissioning in England and other countries

This book does not seek to examine commissioning systems outside England in detail, but the key differences are outlined here. These differences are especially important for English commissioners to understand where their services border these countries geographically. In addition, examination of the different systems highlights the similarities which make up a successful commissioning approach.

Commissioning in Wales

In 1969, legislation was passed moving control of the NHS in Wales to the Welsh Office, a UK government department. Since this time, the Welsh Government has set NHS strategy and ensured delivery of services for the three million people living in Wales.

In Wales, seven local health boards are responsible for the planning and implementation of care in their areas. As well as the main physical health services, this arrangement includes dental, pharmacy, optical, and mental health. There are three NHS Wales trusts with responsibility for public health, ambulance services, and cancer and blood services. Finally, there are two special health authorities operating nationally. Digital Health and Care Wales is responsible for digital solutions for healthcare. Health Education and Improvement Wales is responsible for the Welsh healthcare workforce and covers training, education, and development.

The key difference in commissioning between England and Wales is that Wales doesn't have a purchaser–provider split – that is, commissioners don't buy services from providers; rather, the two functions are combined and operate as one through integrated health boards.

There are cross-border arrangements for those who reside in Wales or England and receive care over the border.

Commissioning in Scotland

The NHS in Scotland is governed by the Scottish Government. There are 14 regional NHS boards, which plan and deliver health services for their communities. This includes protection and improvement of health as well as delivery of frontline services. In addition, there are seven regional special NHS boards and one public health body, all of which support the regional boards. The special NHS boards provide a range of national specialist services; they are Healthcare Improvement Scotland, NHS Education for Scotland, the NHS National Waiting Times Centre, NHS 24, the Scottish Ambulance Service, the State Hospitals Board for Scotland, NHS National Services Scotland, and Public Health Scotland.

In 2022, the Scottish Government proposed legislation to support social care reform. They are suggesting a radical change, with responsibility for health and social care services moving from local authorities to government ministers from 2026. The government will have a new national body – the National Care Service. This will set standards and commissioning priorities for new local care boards. The intention is to drive consistency and improve quality. The format and function are still under development, but this is a very different approach from that in England. Many will be watching to see how this operates and what the outcomes will be.

In this new model, community health and social care boards will replace the existing integration authorities, which are very much like England's integrated care boards. The control of these new boards will be led by national government. There are at present no plans to change the Scottish social care patient payment arrangements whereby individuals receive personal and nursing care free of charge but means testing applies to other services, such as help with housework or shopping.

Like Wales, there are cross-border arrangements between Scotland and England to ensure that people get the care and support they need without confusion or delays.

Commissioning in Northern Ireland

In England, Wales, and Scotland, healthcare is provided by the NHS and social care is provided by local authorities, but with varying levels of collaboration and control. In Northern Ireland, the two are closely combined in the Health and Social Care model.

Health and Social Care is overseen by the Department of Health (one of nine Northern Ireland Executive departments), with the duty of delivery discharged to the Health and Social Care bodies. Currently, these bodies consist of the Strategic Planning and Performance Group within the Department of Health, the Public Health Agency, five local commissioning groups, which cover the same geographical area as five health and social care trusts, and 17 integrated care partnerships (across the five local commissioning group areas). The Northern Ireland Ambulance Service is a sixth trust.

The health and social care trusts provide a range of care services, including acute, mental health, community, and social care services (the latter including nursing home and domiciliary care).

Northern Ireland's integrated care partnerships have many similarities with the integrated care systems in England. They both aim to bring partners together to improve and coordinate care. These structures were established in 2013 and so have been around for longer. The number of people each integrated care partnership serves is relatively small at around 100,000. Therefore, the footprint is similar to a small place or large neighbourhood in England. There was a consultation in 2021 on the future of the these partnerships. This aims to inform the further enhancement of the arrangement, including through improved continuity of care and more empowered communities.

Comparing commissioning in the four countries of the UK

In 2014, the Nuffield Trust and Health Foundation completed a study on the performance of the NHS systems across the four countries of the UK (Bevan et al, 2014). The aim was to see how devolvement and differences in policy had affected performance. Their findings, based on 20 comparable indicators, suggest that the performance and progress made by all four was comparable, with no one country outperforming or doing much worse than the others.

It would be interesting to see this comparison repeated in a few years, once the new integrated care system structure is fully embedded and after other UK countries have made their changes, such as the introduction of the National Care Service in Scotland and the improvements to partnerships in Northern Ireland.

Commissioning outside the UK

I do not attempt to summarise the models of international healthcare systems and how they are governed across the world, but I make the point that there are many learning opportunities out there. These learning opportunities may be for large-scale NHS structural design – for example, through watching the developments and challenges of the new Japanese social care system (see Curry et al, 2018) or, closer to the reach of individual commissioners, the design of health and social care delivery models for disease groups or populations. In these explorations, it is a case of trawling the Internet, academic research, and other sources to see what has been implemented with success elsewhere. It is useful to be curious and innovative when examining these alternatives, but always be mindful of the following:

• Is it safe and effective? If very experimental, you will almost certainly need to test it safely first. Are there differences in national standards or legislation that will prevent its application?

- Will it be accessible to all groups who need it? Are the populations it seeks to serve comparable?
- Are the right skills and workforce available for it? Will it require lengthy training or recruitment programmes?
- Are new premises or specific equipment needed for it?
- How will this work with existing financial systems (how would it be paid for)?

Learning from international health and social care delivery can be presented as options in the commissioning design process, and then, if this option is selected, it can be co-produced, taking account of any local variations required.

The King's Fund reviewed literature on international commissioning models and compared them with those in England (see Anandaciva, 2023). They concluded that the UK was middle of the pack regarding outcomes and resources. They found that no single model of commissioning produced consistently better results than others – all UK countries strive to improve outcomes by developing the model they already have, with very few radical transformations in systems.

REFLECTIONS FOR LEADERS

Integrated care systems and co-production

The new integrated care system structure for the NHS will take time to bed in and there will be challenges. However, there are undoubtably opportunities with the improved conditions for collaboration and co-production. As noted in Chapter 1, good health and wellbeing is not just the absence of illness, but a combination of factors to be approached holistically. Closer working with partners across an area will build stronger foundations for collaboration and, in turn, improve understanding of the opportunities for enhancing positive health, community health, wellbeing, and community resilience.

The approach is not entirely new. Joint strategic needs assessments by clinical commissioning groups and local authorities have been around for some time, but the structure for organisations working together is strengthened within the integrated care system structure, and there is stronger governance in place with the Health and Care Act 2022.

As rosy as this approach sounds, it is at the time of writing a new way of working. This structure requires the dilution of long-standing barriers between commissioners and providers, which will not happen effectively overnight. Getting there will require that system leaders model the new behaviours and enable others to do the same.

Reports influencing local strategy

The **Fuller Stocktake Report** (Fuller, 2022) shares a vision for improving primary care and integrating services for the benefit of people and their communities. It aims to streamline access to care, improve the offer of personalised care approaches, and support people to stay well for longer. These recommendations sit well with the formation of the new integrated care systems and will be a strategic priority for many.

The **Hewitt Review** (Hewitt, 2023) examined the structure of integrated care systems and sought to determine if they have the right conditions to succeed. The review identified key principles that will enable integrated care systems to thrive and deliver. These are:

- collaboration within and between systems and national bodies;

- having a limited number of shared priorities – not trying to do everything, but rather focusing on key areas;

- allowing local leaders the space and time to lead;

- having the right support, balancing freedom with accountability;

- enabling access to timely, transparent, and high-quality data.

Overall, the review was positive. It suggests the integrated care system structure is an opportunity for improvement of health and wellbeing in the future.

Suggestions for success

Relationships are key – get to know your partners and involve them where you can. Yes, they can sometimes create issues, but if they are properly involved, problems will be less likely. In any case, the benefits they bring with their expertise and leadership is worth it.

Although throughout this book I encourage developing and maintaining good relationships, there is a caveat: be wary of becoming too cosy. If relationships are too close, this can make things uncomfortable when problems are tackled. Holding each other to account is still an important duty, and of course professionalism between partners is essential when dealing with challenges together.

4

Using data and intelligence

Aim

The practical advice begins in this chapter, with tools and techniques for identifying local needs – including population health assessment and mapping current provision – and then how to use data and intelligence to inform the commissioning approach. Analysis of data and how to present intelligence are briefly examined.

Understanding population health

Population health

Population health is an approach that aims to improve health and wellbeing outcomes, and reduce avoidable health inequalities. Population health management is a way of working to help health and care agencies understand current health and care needs and predict what local people will need in the future. This supports commissioning approaches that are tailored to better care and support for individuals, create joined-up and sustainable health and care services and make better use of public resources. In summary, population health is about understanding local populations in order to better design services to meet their needs.

Population health analysis uses many different types and sources of information to better understand what factors are affecting health and wellbeing in population groups. Local health and care services can then design and offer models of care and support which will improve health and wellbeing for the local population now as well as for the future. As each population is different, this must be done locally to fully understand specific needs.

To be clear, this is not looking at wide population needs and then clumsily commissioning a catch-all solution, as in 'diabetes admission rates are generally high, so let's commission more diabetes nurses across the whole area'. It is more nuanced and specific than that. For example, diabetes admission rates are higher in South Asian communities (Shah and Kanaya, 2014) and in those with unskilled jobs and those who are unemployed (Kilvert, 2023). New models of working could target these groups in ways that will be effective for them. For example, partnerships involving health services, public health, and communities could offer cooking classes, diet and nutrition advice in workplaces, and free gym memberships for specific groups. It is about using the data to be more proactive and targeted when tackling local issues, to meet people's needs in the best way.

The importance of population health

The principles of good population health assessment are important and should be considered in every large-scale commissioning project. For example:

- Has the cohort of people with most need been accurately identified?
- Are the cohort needs fully understood?
- What other influences are affecting this cohort's health and wellbeing?

By getting into the habit of asking and answering these questions, commissioners can be more assured they are meeting the needs of their population, and therefore more likely to achieve real outcomes.

A fictional example drawing on these questions is provided in Table 4.1.

Table 4.1: Using population health analysis

Example service: Post-treatment support for men who had prostate cancer surgery
Service aim is to improve the health and wellbeing of men post surgery with improved recovery times, reduced follow-ups, and fewer subsequent mental health referrals

---

The question	The analysis
Has the cohort of people with most need been accurately identified?	Analysis of data and intelligence: • 50% of men don't accept the offer of post-treatment support. • Of those who don't accept post-treatment support, 95% are working-age men. Conclusion: • The cohort with greatest unaddressed need is men of working age. Potential solution: • Examine the time of day and days of the week when support is offered and consider weekend or evening programmes.
Are the cohort needs fully understood?	Analysis of data and intelligence: • The post-surgery support offer is predominantly advice on wound care. • The support offer has a rigid structure with no opportunity for peer support. • Surveys of men suggest they want more advice on sexual health. • National research suggests men find it harder to discuss worries and concerns than women. Conclusion: • The current support offer is not fully meeting the needs of men. Potential solution: • Work with men who have experienced prostate surgery to design the post-surgery support offer with the content they need, shared in a way that is helpful and meaningful for them. • Support the development of peer support groups in the community.
What other influences are affecting this cohort's health and wellbeing?	Analysis of data and intelligence: • When examining national datasets, we can see that local recovery times are longer than the national average benchmark, especially in more deprived areas. • Follow-ups with complications are higher in men from deprived areas and from minority ethnic groups. • Fewer men from deprived areas and minority ethnic groups attend a full series of support sessions. Conclusions: • There may be more urgency to return to work for people in lower socioeconomic groups. • Men in deprived areas and from minority ethnic groups may find accessing the post-surgery support more difficult. Potential solutions: • Offer non-health support, such as advice on return to work and support with managing finances. • Ensure that the offer of support is accessible in localities with most need – engage with people to find out how access can be improved regarding place, time, and other barriers, such as cultural and language differences.

A wide-reaching population health assessment won't be necessary for all commissioning projects. Small-scale changes can offer big impacts even when based on a few sources of data, as illustrated in the example. Assessment needs to be proportionate to the scale of the service in question.

Data and intelligence sources

Intelligence is any type of information that gives us insight into what is happening locally, what the needs of a group or population are, and what might work to meet these needs. There are multiple sources of intelligence that can be used to assess population need. Some key types are summarised in Table 4.2. It isn't necessarily the case that all of these are needed in every project, but a cross-section of multiple sources can give a fuller picture.

In addition to data and intelligence, local knowledge and strategic understanding are of benefit to commissioners. The following factors can shape commissioners' output significantly, so they need to be understood in detail:

- local strategy – the solution needs to be in keeping with local priorities or there needs to be a very strong case for change. Local strategic plans usually indicate where any new money will be directed;
- national policies or legalities – if the area of focus is a national priority, this will strengthen the case for change. If it goes against national policy, then it is unlikely to ever get the green light (and there will probably be good reason for this);
- what money is in the system, and its availability – a key question is whether there is funding available to support any changes. If your locality is struggling financially, then unless you have a very strong case for a change, or the solution is free, the answer is likely to be no. This does not mean nothing can be done, but you may have to design a solution within the means available;
- timescales – if the need is urgent, the time to do a full analysis is limited. Sometimes, a quick solution is best followed by a longer review with a full solution implemented later;
- reputation – this shouldn't be a big driving factor but unfortunately it often is. For example, a commissioner may

recommend an unpopular solution, such as decommissioning or reducing a service. The locality leaders may go against this solution on risk to reputation alone. It's worth considering this and how to mitigate against it, usually with a clear case for change;

- other risks – are there other risks associated with the proposed commissioning change? If so, these need to be understood sooner rather than later. They may become a barrier later in the process.

Table 4.2: Sources of data and intelligence

Data/intelligence source	What it can tell you	Things to note
Asset mapping for the locality – details of all the current services already available	This tells you what services are already in place.	This can be more complex than it sounds, as there may be provision in place that you are unaware of, such as by the VCSE or charitable sector. Or, you might find that the services you know are in place aren't delivering the specifics you need. Therefore, you need to be sure what services are available, what they are delivering and for whom, and whether this is being done well. Mapping will also highlight gaps in provision.
Local activity data from providers	Usually, this is quantitative data on what is being provided and to whom. It may also offer information on patient demographics or process data, such as how long people have waited for a service.	Note that this data is not always complete or accurate. Assess the data quality.
Patient outcomes data	Again, this is usually available from providers. This is often quantitative and might include, for example, the number of successful recoveries from surgery or people with improvement in pain.	This data is important as an indicator of success for those who have accessed the service in question.

Table 4.2: Sources of data and intelligence (continued)

Data/intelligence source	What it can tell you	Things to note
Demographic data for the area	This might include local authority population data, such as the number of people in different age brackets or the number of children in care.	This may help with estimating demand for a new approach or identifying unmet need.
Benchmarking data	Benchmarking involves comparing your data with that of others in areas of a similar size or with a similar demographic.	This is useful for gauging what you need and can be valuable for making the case for change.
Best practice models or national guidance	This provides examples of how the problem (or a similar problem) has been addressed with success, and may include recommendations for practice.	This is very useful as the information takes out some guess work, but local variables may affect how it works in your area – adaptations are usually required.
Academic studies	These can analyse the issues and potential effective solutions.	This is useful for understanding and examining large-scale changes.
Financial data	The cost of contracts or costs of services is sometimes available via Patient Level Information and Costing System data, which give you a single cost for a patient's journey through the acute care system, or the social return on investment, which indicates savings from implementing community initiatives.	This is useful for understanding value for money and affordability, and may help demonstrate how doing something different may save money.
Surveys	These can be used to get feedback from the service users, the public, and professionals.	This is a good way to contact large numbers, but surveys always have limitations, such as survey fatigue and respondents not understanding the question.
Interviews, focus groups, and conversations	These data sources offer an in-depth understanding of people's views and experiences.	Conversations with people who have lived experience are especially valuable. These offer a rich source of information but are time-consuming to carry out.

Good to know: What is a patient 'demographic'?

Demographics are statistics that describe populations and their characteristics.

Demographic analysis provides the characteristics of a population, including the age, ethnicity, and sex distributions. Demographic data also include socioeconomic data, related to employment, education, income, marriage rates, birth rates, death rates, and more.

National data sources

There are several national datasets and repositories available for commissioners. NHS England has responsibility for the collection and presentation of these datasets. They are used to inform commissioning decisions and policy, to support monitoring, and to improve care.

The three data sources with the biggest scope are discussed in this section. These all have patient-level data – that is, the data are details about individual patients, including their demographic characteristics, their co-morbidities (diseases and disorders), any treatment or health services contacts they have had, and their medical history. This information is provided anonymously – no names are provided. And they are all 'secondary use' datasets. This means the data are collected by people other than those using them, like clinicians. The data are collected for analysis and research into operational services and patient needs.

The data sources are very useful and robust sources of intelligence. NHS England (2023c) sets out the benefits of this data, noting that it provides:

- national, comparable, standardised data about groups of services that are being delivered, which will support decision making;
- information on the use of resources to improve the operational management of services;

- information on outcomes, to help to address health inequalities;
- visibility of expenditure, allowing the implementation of new payment approaches, such as community currencies or mental health resource groups (see Chapter 7);
- information to improve reference costs for services, to ensure that these are reported consistently and continue to accurately represent costs;
- support for a nationally consistent clinical record for all patients across England, which can be used to support national research projects;
- information for the future development of services.

NHS England aims to reuse clinical data already collected for direct patient care, therefore minimising the burden of data collection overall.

They are mandatory datasets, so providers must submit data on a monthly basis using the SNOMED CT (Systemised Nomenclature of Medicine Clinical Terms) coding system within the electronic patient record. SNOMED CT is a comprehensive collection of clinical terms with associated codes for use in electronic systems. It was developed in the US in 2007 and is used today as a consistent vocabulary for professionals, healthcare providers, and commissioners – it is like a shared language. The electronic data collection must be completed by all publicly funded community, mental health and secondary care services, including the independent sector wherever the defined services are provided.

Community Services Data Set

All types of community services are included in this dataset, but some services of note are health visiting, district nursing, musculoskeletal services, school nursing, community dental services, community paediatrics, speech and language therapy, and weight management services.

The Community Services Data Set is available for use by all, and it is used by commissioners and partners to examine trends. NHS England publish monthly national reports on the website, usually two to three months behind collection, but this is still relatively timely (see https://digital.nhs.uk/data-and-informat ion/data-collections-and-data-sets/data-sets/community-servi ces-data-set).

Figure 4.1 is an example of the type of data that are freely available – it shows the top reasons for referral broken down by age categories.

Mental Health Services Data Set

This dataset is inclusive of all mental health conditions, all support needed for mental wellbeing, learning disabilities, autism, and other neurodevelopmental conditions. All providers of these services must submit data.

Dashboards are available, and these are updated monthly. They have limitations, however, due to incomplete data collection. They can't indicate:

- how many people were in contact with secondary mental health services or subject to the Mental Health Act;
- whether variations are due to the mental illness existing in the population, the service provision, or data quality issues.

The available dashboards are:

- Mental Health Time Series data – this includes key metrics, such as trends of contacts nationally and demographic breakdowns.
- Mental health services – data are specific to providers and/or areas. This is very useful for examination of local data.
- Mental Health Act – this includes data on detentions (sections), community treatment orders or conditional discharge, and short-term detention orders. All of these are Mental Health Act assessment and treatment rights of people with a mental health disorder. The data are available by provider and area.
- Mental health service referrals and care contacts for children and young people – this includes data on referrals, attended contacts, and missed contacts for people aged up to 18 years. The data is available by provider and area.

Figure 4.1: Example of Community Services Data Set monthly statistics

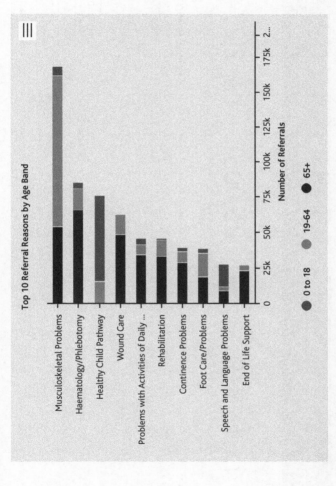

Source: NHS Digital (2023a), Open Government Licence v3.0

Figure 4.2: Example of the Mental Health Services Data Set monthly statistics

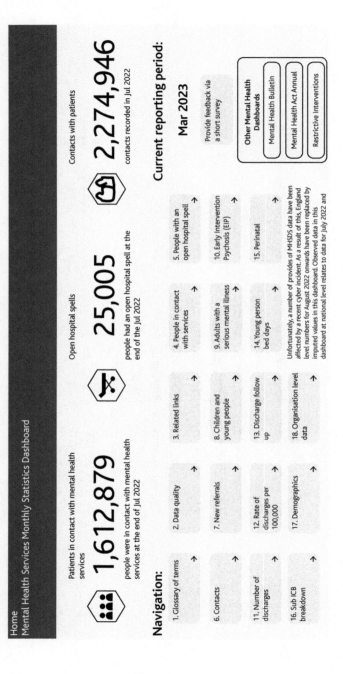

Source: NHS Digital (2023b), Open Government Licence v3.0

(See more at: https://digital.nhs.uk/data-and-information/ data-collections-and-data-sets/data-sets/mental-health-servi ces-data-set)

Figure 4.2 shows an example of the monthly Mental Health Time Series data report. This dashboard gives the number of people in contact with mental health services, the number of active hospital spells, and the total contacts for the month in question. The dashboard provides national data for a range of other aspects of care and quality which commissioners can explore.

Secondary Uses Service repository

This repository includes the data that would have previously been required for the National Tariff (now NHS Payment Scheme). Therefore, it covers acute care (or secondary care) services predominantly. This is a massive data processing system and in 2022 on average it was processing 6 million submitted records per day, and 28 million outbound extracted records per day (NHS Digital, 2023c).

Monthly summaries are not freely available. This data is accessed via a secure portal and with an NHS smartcard (a card that controls access to sensitive data). This process allows permitted commissioners or users to download data extracts to support local summary analysis and reporting. Providers can access patient confidential data, but commissioners can only see pseudonymised records. (See more at: https://digital.nhs.uk/services/secondary-uses-service-sus)

Good to know: Access to sensitive and personal data

The Data Protection Act came into effect in 2018. This legislation ensures that people's data are handled securely and in line with regulations.

Commissioners and NHS England maintain a legal right to collect information – this information is needed to run effective services, plan for the future, manage epidemics, and enable research. However, there are restrictions on what is collected and how it is stored, shared, and used. For example, commissioners do not need to know any details that can identify the individual. These details are removed if it is collected by providers, before it can be used. The data that are made available for use are 'anonymised'. On some occasions, commissioners will need to see some data that could potentially identify individuals – that is, 'identifiable data'. There are very strict rules for the use of this data, and it is only used where absolutely necessary.

'Pseudonymised data' has 'identifiable data' replaced with an artificial identifier or pseudonym. This can protect privacy. For example, your NHS number, postcode, and date of birth can lead to your identification, so the data are replaced with unique codes. Specialist software completes this task, and the process can be reversed if needed for a specific valid reason.

See more on data protection at: www.gov.uk/data-protection

Interpreting data and intelligence

Analysing data and intelligence

For large-scale commissioning projects, commissioners will accumulate a range of sources of intelligence to help them understand the population health and the context they are operating within. Ideally, this data will be in many forms, including **quantitative** (measurable in numbers) and **qualitative** (concepts, meanings, experiences) data. This mix is important, as it allows for a deeper and richer understanding of what is happening (or not happening) locally.

Table 4.3 sets out the broad steps for doing data analysis and sharing key findings. Two approaches to analysis are described next.

Strategic analysis

A strategy is a specific statement about what a system needs to ensure services are in place to meet population health and wellbeing priorities. It usually takes into account a strategic analysis of local intelligence and local and national drivers, to articulate the desired outcomes.

Strategic analysis and a subsequent plan are beneficial because this:

• communicates to all partners, and the public, what the vision and key priorities are;

- is a process usually undertaken with partners and therefore is a joint mission statement, which helps:
  - o partners work more closely together;
  - o integrate provision more effectively;
- provides clear priorities for available funding;
- provides the basis for business plans and investment plans as a source of evidence.

This will provide a clear basis for locally agreed priorities. Then, with partners, the commissioner would formulate options for tackling these priorities. These options would consider timeframes, risks, and costs. The final stage is agreeing the high-level plan as

Table 4.3: Steps for data analysis

1. *Be clear on what you are aiming to understand* – define the parameters of your study; if you cast your data net too wide, you will get lots of information you don't need, and that will slow you down. Make sure your analysis aligns with the question you are trying to answer.

2. *Collect data using a wide range of sources* – where possible, use both quantitative and qualitative data, as these offer different insights.

3. *Clean the data* – remove anything that is not relevant, a duplication, or inaccurate.

4. *Analyse the data to find trends, patterns, and variations* – triangulate all your data sources; that is, compare them to each other to look for patterns and test your findings. You could also triangulate with national policy, legislation, or standards. Where you can, benchmark your findings against data from other areas, especially where there are similarities in population demographics.

5. *Interpret the data* – consider what the data is telling you. There may be more than one interpretation. Try to avoid bias – it is better to have a few people interpreting data. Sharing your key data along with your interpretations will allow others to test your findings. It is fine to make assumptions, but you need to make it clear if that is what you have done. Small research groups may be helpful, but it will depend on the scale of your project.

6. *Clearly present the issues and their impacts* – share the potential impacts of your findings. Even if you don't know with certainty what the impacts will be, you can make some assumptions – for example, people who don't attend cancer screening are at higher risk of needing longer or more extensive treatment when finally diagnosed, and there are potentially preventable deaths.

7. *Present recommendations or options based on your analysis* – set out which aspects need to be tackled. Any recommendations should point out the risks of the suggested option, but also the risks of doing nothing.

a collective. A strategy plan will include funding estimates and timescales, but the granular detail is more likely to be captured in project plans.

Gap analysis

This usually forms part of the analysis process and is the step taken after identifying what the population needs are. The gap analysis helps to explore what commissioners already have in place for tackling the needs they have identified. It addresses the essential question of: where are we now?

Commissioners need to explore the nature, the intent, the offer, and the location of all the relevant services. This includes the services they know about, but it also requires some digging to see if there are other unknown services out there that also address this need. These could be services that are not commissioned by the commissioner's own organisation, such as a local authority-commissioned service (if a health commissioner) or a service provided by a voluntary, community and social enterprise (VCSE) organisation.

The following questions may help the process of gap analysis – keep the identified need in mind as you consider them:

- What gaps are there for services for this need?
- What gaps are there within specific localities, groups of people, and communities?
- How accessible are services regarding referral processes, location, physical access, transport, interpreters?
- Are any of these services weak or poor in quality?
- Is there overprovision of services?
- What are the funding sources, and are these sustainable?
- Are current services sustainable regarding other factors, such as skilled workforce?

Presenting findings

Methods of presenting findings and subsequent recommendations or options are summarised in Table 4.4. There are similarities among the approaches, and you can select an approach to meet

Table 4.4: Presenting data analysis

Method	Approach
Business case	Usually, this takes a predetermined structure setting out context, rationale, evidence, cost, resource implications (for example, for the workforce), timescales, and other details that a board or similar group would need to understand before making a decision. Often, expected outcomes, cost, and risk will be key features of making the case for change.
Options appraisal	This is simply a method of displaying several options alongside each other. You could do this to compare elements such as expected outcomes, cost, workforce, and risks. It provides a summary of what the options could be.
Cost–benefit analysis	This is more specific than options appraisal. Cost–benefit analysis quantifies the costs and benefits of a service or programme in monetary value. Decisions are based on whether benefits are equal to the costs.
Social return on investment	This method incorporates the cost–benefit analysis but applies a wider and more holistic view of value for money. Social return on investment is a framework for measuring and accounting for a much broader concept of value than just monetary value. It incorporates social, environmental, and economic costs and benefits, and helps organisations to better understand the value that they create.
Feasibility study	This assesses the practicalities of a plan. It looks at the probability of success, examining factors such as fit with existing services, funding and resources required, training needs, locations, digital requirements, equipment, and previous applications of the approach elsewhere. It presents key risks and probability of success, but it is also a very useful approach to plan the implementation of a project once agreed.

the particular needs of your project or your local preferences. The findings from data analysis must be presented and shared with decision makers in order to have impact. Table 4.4 summarises some of the approaches for sharing data analysis. Commissioners will choose appropriate methods that are in-keeping with local processes, but also reflect the scale and key messages of the findings. For example, business cases and social return on investment approaches will focus on the value for money and expected outcomes. Option appraisals will support decision making where there are multiple choices. Feasibility studies explore risks and predicted outcomes for operational changes.

Whatever approach is utilised be aware that this data analysis will be an important part of rationale for commissioning change. Therefore, it needs to be clearly presented with limitations of the data analysis included for transparency.

REFLECTIONS FOR LEADERS

Population health: Choosing priorities

Using population health analysis for commissioning can be messy and complex. There will undoubtably be many gaps that require addressing, and it can be confusing and contentious to know what to tackle first and how with often limited resources.

Collaboration is key to working through the competing priorities. Be open and transparent with your partners, and enable conversations where joint leadership decisions are made about where to focus energy and resources. That way, you will likely benefit from people involved in decision making paving the way to more effective change management, and they can also support difficult discussions about what must wait.

You can acknowledge the key gaps that can't be addressed immediately by including them in plans for the longer term, with strategies looking at longer-term goals. You will need to build in flexibility, as priorities will change, but this strategic acknowledgement will be useful for partners to see that they are not forgotten or ignored.

Suggestions for success

Data and intelligence are important elements for commissioning well, but sometimes the sources are scarce, incomplete, or inaccurate. In these circumstances, you may have to use what you have and make some assumptions based on that. This is where your expertise and experience, and that of your partners, comes into play. It is better to start solving a problem on educated guess work rather than wait another year or two for more robust data and have patients miss out on improved care.

It's important, especially for larger commissioning projects or programmes, to test what you think you 'know'. You do this partly with data and intelligence, but it's especially valuable to talk to people who have a good understanding of the area in question. This may be those who deliver services or work with the cohort, or people who are living with the condition or have used similar services. Talking to these groups of people and including them in the process of identifying need is very beneficial, especially where the data is lacking.

Be open and curious in challenging your own views and keep an open mind. Inviting in a range of diverse views is a surer route to implementing successful solutions.

5

Collaborative service design

Aim

This chapter covers the processes and steps to take when designing and delivering service change. Key to success is the application of co-production, so this is described along with tips for how to do it well. The service specification is an important document for commissioning, and it is useful for implementing change, so the chapter looks at how to use that tool. The chapter also outlines some of the important factors affecting operational design, such as capacity and demand planning, workforce, and how to integrate with other services.

Service design approaches

When to commission change

When we talk about commissioning change, we generally refer to large-scale changes – not tweaks to existing services. A service change that requires more robust commissioning usually involves a significant change regarding time or cost required or a very new way of working.

And regardless of scale, there are essentially three circumstances when change is appropriate: when there is a gap in provision; when quality of provision and outcomes are poor; and when it is mandatory (see Table 5.1).

Table 5.1: When to commission change

Situation	Example	Action
Where analysis shows there is a **gap** in provision	People leaving orthopaedic surgery don't have ongoing rehabilitation support.	Commissioners and partners identify effective solutions and commission new provision.
Where analysis shows there is **poor quality or poor outcomes** and opportunity for significant improvement	Data suggest people with diabetes in the locality are not managing their insulin levels well, and emergency admissions are higher than average.	Commissioners and partners identify what needs are unaddressed and either commission new provision or lead service change with existing providers.
Mandated change needs to be coordinated	National guidance suggests community services must link more effectively with primary care.	Commissioners lead multiple providers in designing and implementing change to meet national requirements.

Service design or redesign

Service design can be defined as the activity of planning and organising processes, people, infrastructure, communication, and the components of a service, to improve quality, outcomes, the interaction between the service provider and patients, and patient experience. Good service design is required to effectively meet the local needs of the population, the priorities for health and wellbeing, and it must be sustainable.

If the needs analysis has been completed comprehensively (see Chapter 4), the commissioner will have improved their understanding of local needs and priorities. A gap analysis will have shown what is already available, and they will have a good understanding of the current priorities. The next step is to design change for improvement or to meet any unmet need, and implement this to reach the 'desired state'. These steps are shown in Figure 5.1.

The service design is the approach to address the gaps and reach the desired state. However, commissioners are working within restricted and limited circumstances within the public sector – that

Figure 5.1: Steps to the desired state

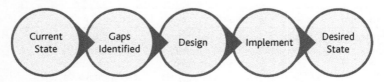

is a challenge that is not going to go away any time soon. They will be limited by:

- what they can afford;
- what resources they can access, such as workforce, premises, equipment;
- what expertise they have available, such as skills in service design.

These factors will steer what can ultimately be achieved. For these reasons, it is difficult to provide step-by-step guidance or detailed models. However, to inspire planning, the following options can be considered:

- expansion – simply providing more of what is already working well to meet more demand;
- improvement additions – providing 'bolt-on' improvements to an existing service and leaving the majority as it currently operates;
- 'fresh start' redesign – taking an old service and redesigning how the whole service operates;
- innovation – designing a totally new approach that may require some testing – you can bolt this on to existing services, or it can be part of a 'fresh start' redesign;
- integration – working alongside other providers/services to offer an integrated service rather than silo working. This approach can share resources and reduce the number of hand-offs between services, thereby improving the patient experience;
- changing specific factors such as:
  o location – providing care closer to home or in the home;
  o method of delivery – face to face or virtual;
  o personalised care approach (see Chapter 10);

    o   access to services – for example, changing referral processes or targeting populations.

These can be used individually or in combination. For all of them, service design often will have a specific approach, which may be:

- an outcome-focused approach – focuses on the impact of the service on an individual's health and wellbeing outcomes rather than on productivity, such as number of procedures performed;
- a pathway approach – focuses on the individual's journey through the service and how to provide accessible and easy-to-use services with a clear pathway from beginning to end from the individual's perspective;
- a whole-system approach – cuts across organisational boundaries and clinical disciplines aiming for seamless transfers or shared care. It has the potential for pooling resources and reducing duplication to provide seamless care for individuals.

There is a tendency in service design for organisations to tweak historic arrangements, with small incremental changes over time. Radical change is rarer and often more difficult to implement. However, due to the increasing focus on health inequalities, the impact of the COVID-19 pandemic, and the greater pressure for efficiencies in recent years, many have been forced to review their services on a grander scale, and it has brought a new urgency to identify what services to commission, for whom, and how best they can be delivered. Both small incremental change and radical large-scale change can be the right thing to do depending on the circumstances.

Redesign for incumbent services

An incumbent service is a service which is already being provided. In reality, most service design is based on this position of a provider already in place providing a service which could be improved or changed to meet needs better or more fully.

    This starting position should not significantly affect the design process. The possible scenarios for improvement include those mentioned earlier, such as expansion or improvement additions, and can even include fresh start redesign depending on the scale of change needed.

Relationships with providers must be handled with care. It is important that they are involved in the process of identifying the need for change and that they are partners in developing the solutions. The exception to this rule is where there are significant changes that may involve procurement processes, as in fresh start approaches. Here you need to be mindful of procurement rules. (Chapter 6 provides more detail on how to manage these changes through contracting processes.)

Phases of service design

For simplicity, the key activities of service design can be broken down into four key stages:

1. Pre-design and vision.
2. Design for the desired state.
3. Testing of the approach.
4. Implementation.

Each of these stages are summarised in Table 5.2, providing a steer on how to approach them.

Project planning underpins all four stages. Good project planning identifies the key tasks to be done and who will do them. Milestones are a good way of grouping tasks and assigning endpoints. Commissioners should estimate the time and resources required, be realistic, and factor in potential delays, such as the need for formal sign-off at monthly board meetings. Time should be built in for reviewing progress.

Where there is benefit, commissioners can support the plan and smooth running of the process with protocols and guidelines. Terms of reference for working groups are a good example.

Financial resources and their effect on service design

It is important to understand what exists locally for funding and resourcing service design. There is often a lack of commitment and enthusiasm from commissioners and partners when finances

Table 5.2: Key activities for design stages

Stage	Key activities
1. Pre-design and vision	**Creating the vision** It is important to be very clear what it is you are aiming to do. • What is it you want to achieve as an outcome? • Who will be benefiting? • What are the underpinning values (for example, improving quality or experience)? • Why is this important? This tells people why it is a priority to spend time and resources on your project. If you get this right at the beginning, it will serve as a helpful reminder throughout the process and keep you and your partners focussed on the 'why'. The vision needs to be clear so everyone can understand it and it should be co-produced with those who will be affected by it, including those providing and receiving the eventual service. If these people are part of the process for creating the vision, you are more likely to have effective cooperation and a more effective solution. Effective visions have the following key characteristics (Kotter, 1996): • **Imaginable** – they convey a clear picture of what the future will look like. • **Desirable** – they appeal to the long-term interests of those who have a stake in the outcome. • **Feasible** – they contain realistic and attainable goals. • **Focused** – they are clear enough to provide guidance in decision making. • **Flexible** – they allow the use of initiative and alternative responses in changing conditions. • **Communicable** – they are easy to communicate and can be explained quickly. To create your vision, I would suggest you gather key partners together; they will probably have been involved in the data and intelligence exercises previously and will have contributed to examining the findings and identifying the needs and the gaps. Facilitate partners to the agreement of the vision. If you and your partners are being too ambitious, you may need to break the overall vision down into phases with key milestones – remember the six key characteristics mentioned earlier to help keep focus. Write the vision down in language everyone can understand and agree on. This is the impact or benefit for people and at this stage not what the service will look like.

(continued)

Table 5.2: Key activities for design stages (continued)

Stage	Key activities
	Identifying the risks and opportunities It is a good idea to be clear about potential barriers, risks, and other issues before you get into the detail of design. For example, what is the funding situation? Are there recruitment shortages? Is it politically sensitive? Identifying these in advance can steer your thinking and help avoid disappointment later. Remember the vision must be feasible. On the optimistic side, be aware of any current opportunities – for example, a national steer from NHS England, such as programme working to support the NHS Long Term Plan. They may have an offer of support which focuses on your intended project. Grab what help you can.
2. Design for desired state	**Design process** At this point you can start to explore the options and opportunities for designing the change to achieve your vison. This may take the form of an options appraisal which is then refined to a chosen model, usually through consensus of a working group with multiple partners. Consider the types and approaches to service design applicable to your aims. For each identified option, consider the potential impact, both good and bad, and identify risks or barriers and chances of success. Cost will be an important factor but so is availability of skilled workforce, premises, and equipment. In addition, consider what the impact of change will be – in simple terms, will the outcomes be worth any upheaval and change process? Get this agreed model or approach down on paper and where possible use diagrams. The clearer you can make it at this stage the better, but often there will be unknowns that will have to be worked through later. Try to maintain some flexibility where it may benefit. This is the 'desired state'.
3. Testing the approach	Once you have the key components of the service design agreed in principle, it is time to test these ideas out. This can take several forms and will depend on the scale of the change. Larger or complex changes may require more testing. Here are three methods of testing to consider. **Consultation and engagement** You will probably have formed the model through your working group, but you can, and should, take the proposal to wider consultation and engagement. This will include other professionals and the public.

Table 5.2: Key activities for design stages (continued)

Stage	Key activities
	For this process, clearly set out what the vision is, why it's important, and how you have designed change to achieve this. Be clear on what this may mean and how you will see it working. Be transparent on what the downsides might be. Make sure that those who are potentially affected by the change have meaningful opportunities to share their views – for example, establish focus groups so people can be heard.
	Scenario testing
	A well-designed scenario test, though not as thorough as a pilot, can give an improved understanding of how a service may run in reality. This is a good option when a pilot is too costly or complex, or when the changes it would introduce are not reversible.
	This can be desk-based or involve role-playing with the key providers (including clinicians, administrators, and managers) and fictitious patients, walking through the proposed changes step by step. This can test out the processes but also give confidence to those who will be delivering the change. They will have the chance to ask questions and confirm protocols.
	Testing in practice
	You can thoroughly test out a model using a pilot approach. This allows you to see the service in practice. However, this is not always an option due to time and cost constraints. Testing a smaller component of the change, or confined testing within a smaller cohort or environment, can give good understanding of how a large-scale change may operate.
	This approach allows you to understand what is required to run the service and identify any unknown issues. A pilot phase allows you to address issues before a service is widely applied.
4. Implementation	**Implementation planning**
	When you have adequately tested your model, you can proceed to plan implementation with any applicable modifications. Don't underestimate the complexity of this stage of the process. There are many factors to consider – recruitment, training, change management processes, equipment, premises, IT systems, and much more. Comprehensive project planning with flexibility is key to effective implementation.

(continued)

Table 5.2: Key activities for design stages (continued)

Stage	Key activities
	Implementation in action If there is any perceived risk with implementation, then this should be very closely managed. In these instances, there should be a contingency plan for quickly reinstating the old methods or alternatives if needed. Consider risk and impact on other organisations and be open to identifying unintended consequences quickly. Don't forget to include how you will ensure the aims of the change have been met. Implement processes and systems for effective evaluation. This may include IT systems, new data collection, and training. A defined implementation timescale is important, and the key partners can meet at identified points to assess progress and work through teething problems. Support for providers is essential to ensure that the change meets the objectives successfully. All partners need to maintain a sense of ownership, even at this stage, especially where change is largely untested or has many unknowns. There may be a need to introduce unplanned modifications during implementation. An approach for rapid decision making should be established in advance, in readiness for this.

are in short supply, and a situation where there is 'no new money' may seem like a dead end but it doesn't have to be. Understanding this does not mean that nothing can be done is important – as is persuading others that there are still options available. The financial positions and opportunities are summarised in Table 5.3, starting with the most optimistic.

Good to know: NHS Long Term Plan

The NHS Long Term Plan was introduced in 2019 (NHS England, 2019c). It was developed in partnership with a range of people, including frontline workers, patients and their families, and other experts. It is a five-year plan that aims to incorporate learning from the successes of social commitment and also takes account of concerns about funding, staffing, and inequalities as well as optimism about opportunities for continuing advancement and better care outcomes.

Table 5.3: Change options in relation to funding

Financial position	Opportunities for change
Very large funding pot This may seem like a daydream, but this occasionally happens when something is a key priority or funds have been earmarked to kick-start some major change – an example of this may be investment to deal with priorities during the COVID-19 pandemic.	This is a great opportunity to design and try something large-scale where benefits are likely to outweigh the implications of change. Bear in mind whether or not funds are recurrent (available on an ongoing basis).
New funding (ideally recurrent) The values may vary regarding the proportion of the overall costs, but this is a great start position for any commissioning priority.	This is an opportunity to look at change opportunities such as expansion of an existing service, starting something new, alternative workforce models, or other new ways of working within the available budget.
Non-recurrent funding Non-recurrent means it is time limited. This may be a one-off pot of money, or it may be recurrent for a defined period but will then end.	Although this may seem limiting, it is a good opportunity to 'pump-prime' change – that is, support long-term change that may have one-off funding requirements, like training staff, buying equipment, or providing short-lived initiatives such as targeted screening. You can also consider using the funds to pilot a new approach. Staff can be employed on fixed-term contracts and the service can be evaluated. This evaluation can evidence impact for patients and potentially some cost savings, which can be used as a business case for long-term recurrent funding.
Existing funding only This usually means you must work with what funding is available already. There is no 'new' money.	This lack of new funds does not have to mean that change can't happen. Indeed, it is often when facing these restrictions that innovation is employed well. There are opportunities to do things differently without it costing more money and often there are identifiable cost efficiencies that may release funds (more on this in Chapter 7). An example would be integrating with other services to save some back office costs or to streamline pathways.
Reduction in existing funding This is hopefully rare where you have local needs identified, but it does happen where an organisation is financially struggling or where funding has been shown to be higher than average – for example, where benchmarking has shown your organisation spends more on this need than areas with a similar demographic profile.	In this scenario, you can employ the activities mentioned earlier to seek service efficiencies. And if benchmarking has revealed you spend more than average, then examine what other areas are doing. Can you replicate what works well elsewhere and save money? In this situation, and indeed for all service change, involving patients and communities in designing effective solutions can be very effective.

This document, and any that replace it, is a blueprint for commissioners, providers, and partners, as it sets out the key priorities that should be a driver for change at local level. Where a service design aim is included in the NHS Long Term Plan, this is a powerful justification for change and very difficult to argue against.

The NHS Long Term Plan priorities include:

- a new model for healthcare including:
  - o improving out-of-hospital care and removing the divide between primary and community services;
  - o reducing pressure on emergency hospital services;
  - o giving people more control over their own health and greater access to personalised care;
  - o putting greater focus on population health;
- greater focus on prevention and inequalities;
- greater focus on outcomes, including for:
  - o children and young people;
  - o major health conditions such as cancer and diabetes;
- workforce improvements and support;
- digital-enabled care;
- financial stabilisation.

There was discussion in 2022 regarding a refresh of the plan; however, at the time there was a general consensus that with the pandemic aftermath and the formation of the integrated care systems, commissioners had enough on their plate. There may be a refresh or a replacement in the coming years.

Co-production

I have not been able to find a satisfactory definition of co-production for health and wellbeing, mainly because the definitions seem to focus on co-production with the public as the key definer and do not emphasise contributions from clinicians, local government agencies, community leaders, and so on. I believe true co-production includes all parties. With co-production, commissioners are actively involving people who are experts in the processes of understanding and improving care and support.

The right partners will be able to contribute meaningful intel to the understanding and design of services. I believe that it should include people who use services, clinicians, community leaders, and any others who have a good understanding of the issues faced. They will know what matters and what works. Furthermore, once implemented they will be allies in implementation and socialising the new changes.

Co-production is not just about talking to people. Done well it is a meaningful partnership that affects real change. The Social Care Institute for Excellence share precursors for co-production success, which also represent what makes co-production an effective relationship (Social Care Institute for Excellence, 2022). I offer an adaptation of these key features:

- Define people who access care and support as people with skills.
- Break down the barriers between care recipients and support and professionals.
- Build on people's existing capabilities.
- Include reciprocity (where people get something back for putting something in) and mutuality (people working together to achieve shared objectives).
- Work with peer and personal support networks alongside professional networks.
- Facilitate services by helping organisations to become agents for change rather than just service providers.
- Include community leaders, who know their community well – this might be religious leaders, voluntary, community and social enterprise (VCSE) sector organisations, and public groups with a local interest.

An additional benefit of co-production is that the approach fosters good relationships between commissioners, providers, and people receiving care. It strengthens trust and empowers people to see themselves as part of the solution rather than being 'done to'.

Co-production with the public

'Voices of lived experience' refers to those people who have had, or have, a particular condition or challenge that you are examining for improvement. Or they may be someone close to those affected, such as a parent or a spouse. Just like clinicians and other professionals, they are experts. They can tell you what is needed, what works and doesn't work, but also what really matters to people.

Identifying people, or groups, with voices of lived experience is the first step in the process of co-production with the public. This is easier in some areas of health and social care than others. For example, there will probably be stroke support groups or similar in abundance, along with willing volunteers, but commissioners may struggle to get the interest of people for conditions affecting younger people. You may have to think outside of the box to get meaningful connection with some groups, especially those deemed underserved or seldom heard. Talking to community leaders is often an effective way of learning how to engage with different groups.

Good to know: Underserved and seldom-heard groups

The terms 'underserved' and 'seldom-heard groups' refer to people who are generally under-represented – they tend to be less likely to be heard by the people delivering and designing health services. These groups are sometimes referred to as 'hard to reach'. This term is now outdated, as it suggests that there is something that prevents their engagement with services and that it is the fault of those groups. The terms underserved or seldom-heard emphasise the responsibility of decision makers to reach out to excluded people, ensuring that they have access to engagement and collaboration, and that their voices are heard.

The Healthwatch (2020) guide to co-producing with seldom-heard groups provides examples of these groups:

- ethnic minority groups;
- carers;
- people with disabilities;
- lesbian, gay, bisexual, transgender, and queer people;
- refugees and asylum seekers;
- people who are homeless;

• younger people;
• people with language barriers.

These people may have certain needs when it comes to participating in co-production activities. The general principles of good co-production will apply, but more careful consideration of the following may support effective engagement with these groups:

• Treat people with respect and value all contributions.
• Consider an advocate or a spokesperson who can either speak for a group of people or champion others to get involved.
• Ensure people are very clear about what they can expect if they get involved – and be explicit about what they are expected to contribute or help with.
• Offer a variety of activities and ways to get involved, such as helping others, learning, and socialising, and include different times and places.
• Allocate sufficient resources for communication, transport, meetings, and covering people's costs.

Implementing co-production

When you have identified the people who you need to speak too, a structured approach will be helpful. The Coalition for Personalised Care (2023) offers practical steps to enable meaningful co-production:

• Explain the partnership approach and ensure people understand that they are respected and have an equal voice to commissioners and professionals – try to build a 'level playing field' approach to nurture emerging relationships. In this scenario, they are the experts.
• Use plain language and simple terms; avoid jargon. Ensure people understand the issues.
• Be clear on what the focus of the work is – be open and transparent about what is in scope to change.
• Talk to people in the community or setting of their choice rather than asking them to come to you. The environment is an important part of creating an equal relationship.

- Consider enabling a group of people with similar interests to come together. People often feel more comfortable as part of a smaller group of peers.

And I would add:

- Consider all stakeholders who can influence and shape the service design. Talk to those delivering services already or those who work closely with the people affected.

Co-production on a budget

With the commissioning landscape increasingly restricted regarding capacity and funding, there is the possibility that sometimes co-production efforts will be limited. This can be especially so for engagement and collaboration with underserved or seldom-heard populations as to engage with them effectively may need dedicated time and resources. But this does not mean that it cannot happen at all – co-production can be done well on a shoestring if well planned. Communication and engagement leaders have a variety of resources and methods available to them today. The following are a few ideas of how co-production can be done with very little cost and resource – indeed time and communication are the key factors common to these options.

- Utilise the social media networks that are available and open to all who have access to the Internet – these can be effective routes to seek feedback on surveys or to invite people to events in a local area.
- Use existing groups that will be meeting regularly – this may include general practice public participation groups, support groups, parent governor forums, scouting groups, church gatherings, and so on – maximise these opportunities by asking for an invitation to share your projects and ask for help with feedback.
- Build effective relationships with community leaders – they can act as conduits for your messaging and can help you gain the trust and engagement of underserved or seldom-heard groups.

- Seek to identify passionate volunteers – people with lived experience or their loved ones can often be valuable partners in seeking the wider views of others.
- When designing surveys, keep them succinct and focused on the key areas of interest. Free text boxes can ensure people have the chance to share views on other areas, but the simplified survey will be easier and quicker for a small team to analyse.

Co-production with clinicians

Clinicians are a major influence. Their voices of skilled experience bear a lot of weight with not only those who will be delivering services, but also those who will be funding them. They bring with them a wealth of knowledge of the strengths and weaknesses of the systems to be improved. They can help shape change that is sensible, safe, and effective. And they will know about any applicable professional bodies, standards, or policy. Furthermore, as respected professionals, they will help you land the change more successfully. Their voice will be persuasive when planning and implementing change processes.

There will often be clinicians who 'resist' and are critical of change. This can be for many reasons. However tempting it may be to exclude these people, they should be involved where possible. They can offer alternative perspectives on risks and pitfalls, and if they are persuaded to cooperate and agree to an approach, they can be powerful allies to convince others who have doubts.

Tips for successful engagement with clinicians include:

- Use your agreed vision – this reminds everyone what they are trying to achieve and why. Commissioners can have an unfair reputation of just seeking to cut costs, so show this is not the case.
- Focus on outcomes and values, not targets.
- Be well informed, and use facts and figures you have collected to back up your arguments.
- Use examples of how change has worked well elsewhere – patient stories can be powerful.
- Actively listen and take note of what they have to say; take action on risks and issues that are raised.

- Get to know the clinicians – engage individually rather than as a group if that is helpful – meet at times convenient to them.
- Have a well-prepared project plan with clear objectives.
- Communicate regularly and keep them informed.

In addition to the senior clinical leaders, such as matrons or consultants, don't forget other frontline staff. They are the ones who will actively implement change, so they are important. Keep them involved and informed where possible and ensure their voices are heard. Securing a representative or two in the commissioning processes may be an approach to take for a large body of workforce; or you could join their team meetings to foster a relationship with this often-overlooked group.

Planning and evaluating co-production in commissioning

For robust and effective co-production, consider the following steps for planning and evaluating the approach:

- Include co-production activities, and the time and resources required for them, in your project plan.
- Consider nominating a lead person to coordinate co-production.
- Keep reviewing how well the approach to co-production is working. Is it truly a partnership approach? Are you listening to what is being said? Is co-production making a difference?
- Plan how and when to show people how their contribution has made a difference. Ensure they know they were listened to and that it made an impact.

Community assets

Community assets are anything that can be used to improve community quality of life, health, and wellbeing. They are the essential aspects of community life that bring people together and provide a sense of place. They can include:

- local people and their skills, knowledge, and social networks;
- local groups and social activities;
- local leaders in religion, education, workplaces;

- VCSE organisations;
- buildings and facilities;
- transport networks;
- parks and green spaces.

All these assets can be considered throughout the commissioning cycle. They can potentially contribute through all stages of the cycle.

- Strategic analysis – talking to people and community groups can provide a source of information about people's needs and gaps in services.
- Design – support successful design and effective change via consultation on plans.
- Procure – they can empower local people and community groups to use their abilities to transform the community and support each other. Examples can include community groups to support people with specific needs, such as loneliness.
- Evaluate – they can give feedback on how well a service is working and suggest improvements.

Identifying and mapping community assets is often helpful and sometimes pivotal when designing change. Commissioners can harness the benefits listed here but they can also support the sharing of information about these assets so that more people can benefit from them. Place-based partnerships are often the key link between community assets and more formal health and care services. They are well placed to form effective relationships with communities.

Voluntary, community, and social enterprise sector providers

Community assets, in the form of VCSE organisations, can provide direct services or support. These can range from small community initiatives, such as a social knitting club or a walking group, to larger charitable providers, such as those for long-term conditions or local hospices.

VCSE providers are an important partner for health and social care. They play a significant role in improving health and wellbeing.

National strategy documents reflect this importance. For instance, the VCSE sector is incorporated within the NHS Long Term Plan.

To maximise the benefits of working with VCSE providers, commissioners can take note of the following best practice:

- Notify and involve VCSE partners as early as possible with intentions for planning, design, and delivery – this will increase the chances of these small enterprises having the capacity to effectively collaborate.
- Develop frameworks for commissioning – formally design structures to support the equal partnership approach of VCSE involvement.
- Identify any barriers to VCSE providers playing an equal role, and address them – for example, consider offering a small budget to cover costs of attending meetings.
- Consider joint working – where can VCSE organisations support existing services, and how can they integrate?
- Consider co-funding – share funding of the VCSE sector across multiple partners, all of which would benefit from intervention of the VCSE sector.
- Enable national charities to support local charities – harness their expertise.
- Explore innovative contracting arrangements – can you top-slice a historical contracting arrangement with a large NHS provider to encourage working with the VCSE sector? For example, a community services provider might use 3 per cent of their budget to work with VCSE providers that support the incumbent services effectively.
- Provide sustainability – a VCSE provider that is promised one year of funding may struggle to retain staff or plan for the longer term. Try to agree funding that reflects long-term strategies but has flexibility for some variation year on year.
- Create a single point of access to improve uptake and access. For example, a social prescribing service (more in Chapter 10) can assess people's needs and then match the person to available provision from a local directory. Mapping of all VCSE assets can be undertaken at frequent intervals.
- Consider opening access to NHS or local authority training provision. This can ensure the VCSE workforce have the

necessary skills and knowledge of the wider system and its key working policies, such as safeguarding.

VCSE sector involvement in commissioning

In 2021, NHS England shared a model for supporting the involvement of the VCSE sector in the new integrated care systems (NHS England, 2021a). The aim of the model is to embed VCSE partnership in the integrated care systems including involvement in governance structures, population health management, service redesign, leadership, and organisational development plans.

Essentially, the model advocates VCSE involvement at every level of the system, such as system, place, and neighbourhood. It recognises the need for VCSE collaboration at every tier but with significant involvement in local neighbourhood and/or place communities, as they understand local need and recognise local opportunities.

Embedding VCSE partners at neighbourhood and place levels can be highly effective for targeted collaboration. At neighbourhood level, this could look like involvement in primary care multidisciplinary teams, or links via social prescribing schemes to local activities and services for practical and emotional support. At place level, they could link in with councils or boroughs for planning and delivery. They could also bring their expertise and understanding to health and wellbeing boards for improved locality planning.

VCSE involvement is also valuable at integrated care system level, but as there may be many VCSE bodies, it can become more challenging to get the balance right. To manage this challenge, NHS England recommend an alliance of VCSE bodies for each integrated care system. This is the VCSE health and wellbeing alliance model. The model aims to coordinate collaboration between VCSE bodies and the planners and deliverers of health and care. With this alliance arrangement, the VCSE bodies as a combined body can have a stronger voice to influence commissioning. This can include meaningful representation to the strategic integrated care board and any integrated care system workstreams which affect multiple places. Furthermore, the alliance can facilitate VCSE bodies supporting each other. This could include practical delivery or joining up to share efficiencies at scale.

Commissioners can support the implementation and improvement of VCSE sector alliances with the following actions where an alliance is not yet established:

- Talk to VCSE bodies and identify any barriers to forming an alliance approach – can these be addressed?
- Identify potential leaders who can lead the implementation of an alliance.
- Provide operational support with identifying premises, suggested structures, and example terms of reference or agendas.
- Ensure a VCSE alliance is a clear priority for the integrated care systems and include it in strategic plans.

And where an alliance is established:

- Ensure clear accountability and aims for the alliance are in place, and make sure the alliance is included on integrated care system structures.
- Have identified VCSE representatives attending the integrated care system board and workstreams.
- Have mechanisms in place to ensure information is cascaded effectively to all VCSE bodies.
- Consider funding representatives' time to attend meetings.
- Offer support for self-evaluation of their structure and approach – is it working well for all?

Commissioning VCSE organisations as providers

The majority of VCSE provision takes place without any financial contribution or instruction from commissioners. However, sometimes it can be a viable option to financially support or formally commission them. This may be in full or in part and this usually applicable to larger VCSE arrangements, such as those led by charities, and not for community initiatives, such as peer groups.

Provision from this sector may seem like a cost-effective way of getting what is needed, as they usually provide services for less cost than NHS or independent providers, due to the contribution of charitable funds and the good will of volunteers. However, this should not be seen as an easy option for commissioners. For example, the potential impact of a VCSE may not be able to match that of a service which has greater resources and more expertise; and there may questions regarding quality, safety, productiveness, and sustainability. That is why it is rarely appropriate to entirely replace a formally commissioned and fully funded service with VCSE provision, though this can be done where assurances are in place and a full NHS standard contract is agreed.

As many of the larger VCSE providers are on grant arrangements and not NHS contracts (see more in Chapter 6), there are limits to what governance a commissioner can apply. The solutions for ensuring effectiveness, quality, and safety vary from arrangement to arrangement. Some options to consider for larger VCSE arrangements include:

- grant versus contract – use a contract where the value or volume of activity suggests it will be worth the extra administration time or where there is greater identified risk – this will give improved protection and the VCSE provider will have clear governance frameworks to work within. For example, any funding arrangement above £100,000 could be offered a shorter-form contract (see Chapter 6);
- outcome measures – with all arrangements, be very clear on what the expected outcomes or outputs are, and include this in the written agreement. Outcomes are the benefits realised by an action or series of actions. Outputs are the activities and steps taken. Agree how these will be demonstrated in a proportionate but meaningful way. For example, for a VCSE body receiving a grant for offering support to young people waiting for a mental health assessment, the outcome expectation is that the young people self-report feeling supported and that they receive the information they need 90 per cent of the time or more. Surveys can be used here, and these can be designed to elicit simple data that is easy to collect and interpret;
- risk – where there is an identified risk, agree in advance how this risk will be managed if it occurs. Have this in writing. This will protect people receiving the service but also those delivering

the service. For example, a walking football group receives a small grant and accepts referrals from a social prescribing scheme (see Chapter 10). Some of the people referred may have health risks – for example, they are recovering from a cardiac event. Having a clear protocol in place about action to take in the event of an emergency ensures greater safety for the participants, peace of mind for commissioners and referrers, and confidence and assurance for those providing the activity;

- financial sustainability – if a VCSE provider is offering a service which is usually funded by the NHS (and usually provided by an NHS provider), they need to be sustainable. If not, there is a high risk to continuity of essential services. An example of this situation is charitable hospice care. Hospices often provide a mix of what are traditionally NHS services (inpatient beds or home care with nurses) and traditionally non-NHS services (support groups and complementary therapies). If a hospice is providing traditional NHS services that cannot be provided elsewhere, they need to be supported financially to ensure continuity, safety, and effectiveness. This is often difficult for financially challenged commissioners, but where a hospice is providing essential capacity or services, the commissioner should aim to put in place formal commissioning arrangements. A contract and funding for the core NHS elements will provide sustainability and peace of mind for commissioner and the provider;

- data collection – it is often the case that VCSE providers are either unable or unwilling to collect and share good-quality data. This may be for a variety of reasons, such as feeling at threat of losing money where data shows low productivity; not having the skills, knowledge, or resources for data collection; fear of breaching data protection rules; or feeling the burden of data collection is too great without compensation. To combat this:

  - Ask providers of a similar type or geography to collaborate and work together on improving data collection – this approach can pool resources and focus support provided by commissioners.
  - Provide simple written guidance or workshops to upskill and improve confidence; offer templates for documents such as data sharing agreements.
  - Develop a single-capture system that many providers can input to, with commissioners having the responsibility of

maintaining and ensuring governance – this can also be a vehicle for data sharing across providers who may see the same patient and will benefit from shared care records.

The service specification

The service specification is a document which sets out the key requirements of a service which has been commissioned. It is a document used within the NHS standard contract but can be used in other written agreements too. (I discuss types of contracts more fully in Chapter 6.)

The service specification is helpful because it:

- outlines what a service looks like, how it operates, and who for;
- sets out clearly what the expectations are for both commissioner and provider;
- sets out core standards and those required for ensuring effectiveness, equality, and safety;
- is a record against which provision can be measured and evaluated;
- can be used for procurements, so all bidders are competing for the same set of requirements;
- can set out development requirements.

Types of service specification

In most instances, a service specification is written as part of the service design process. A co-produced service specification will set out what the final design is, how it will operate, and for whom. In some instances – for example, in a procurement exercise – a commissioner may write most of the specification without input from partners, due to competition rules. This is because the rules aim to ensure that no single provider has an unfair advantage over others, but even in these circumstances, the design will be based on conversations that have been held with partners.

Most specifications can be classified into two categories:

- output-based specifications – here, the model and how it will operate is set out in full. The specified process is a priority. The specification is very clear with lots of detail on how, who, where, and so on. This is usually a rigid approach with little or no flexibility for the provider in how it can be delivered. Success is measured by assessing outputs, such as numbers of patients receiving care or the activities completed. It is a useful approach where managing activity and cost is a high priority or where specific standards must be met;

- outcome-based specifications – in these specifications, the outcomes are the priority. The anticipated outcomes for people are specified. 'How' the provider achieves them is for the provider to decide. It is a lot more flexible and can allow the provider to be innovative in how they provide a service to achieve the desired outcomes. It still includes any legislation or relevant standards that must be adhered to.

Generally, the preferred approach is the hybrid approach. A high-level model design can be outlined in a specification, but the details are left to the provider, who will have skills and knowledge for the patient group. The evaluation will then be largely based on pre-agreed measures of outcomes and patient experience. Funding is usually linked to achieving outcomes and/or is a block payment arrangement, with the provider having the freedom to spend it as they see fit to achieve the outcomes.

Components in the service specification

The service specification template provided by NHS England is not mandatory, and commissioners may use their own layout if they wish. However, many continue to use the template, as it is a recommended and well-known approach. It has in recent years been reduced from a larger number of sections to only five. These are shown in Table 5.4 along with some additional sections which may be helpful.

What about capturing evaluation measures and data collection? If the NHS standard contract is used correctly, evaluation measures should be recorded in the relevant separate schedule. There is no need to duplicate. However, for clarity and completeness they can be added to the service specification, especially where there is a team that the specification affects who may not have easy sight of the full contract. Make it work for you.

Table 5.4: NHS standard contract service specification template

Specification section	Explanation	Example
Service name	Be clear in the title **what** it is for and **who** it is for.	Supported self-management for adults with type 2 diabetes.
Service specification number	This is useful if you have many specifications in one contract.	
Population and/or geographical area to be served	Include who is it for and what area it serves.	People aged 18 and over with a diagnosis of type 2 diabetes who reside in Doncaster.
Service aims and desired outcomes	This is usually a clear list of both service aims and expected outcomes.	Aims: • Improve the offer of self-management for people with type 2 diabetes. • Improve access and uptake of the education programmes. • Improve the knowledge, skills, and confidence of people self-managing their condition. Outcomes: • lower recorded Hb1A insulin levels at annual review; • reduced emergency admissions; • improvement in patient reported experience.
Service description and location(s) from which it will be delivered	This is where most of the service detail will go. To help separate some of these details, consider the additional sections below. Locations of service delivery are included here. Locations can be important if targeting particular cohorts. If specified, then a provider cannot move the services without pre-agreement.	Details including the model or pathway plus any applicable standards, such as personalised care approaches. Here you can include eligibility criteria.

(continued)

Table 5.4: NHS standard contract service specification template (continued)

Specification section	Explanation	Example
Additions to consider		
Local and national context	Outline why this service is important, and share the local (and sometimes national) case for the service.	• Summary of the analysis of local needs and any relevant local strategy or policy. • Any national directives, policy, or guidance that has driven this – for example, the NHS Long Term Plan.
Interdependencies with other services	This section is useful for covering the working relationships between organisations and services.	• sharing care records with primary, community, and acute care services; • sharing care clinics between acute and community services; • referral or discharge processes; • links with VCSE organisations.
Applicable national standards	It may be helpful to list national standards here.	National Institute for Health and Care Excellence guidelines and Care Quality Commission requirements.
Date of review	If agreed as applicable, or part of a pilot or testing phase, then a clear date of review can be helpful.	One-year post-start date is commonly used but any relevant period that has been pre-agreed can be entered.

Writing the service specification

The author

Ideally service specification writing should be led by someone with the relevant skills and experience. There is usually a skilled person in most contracting teams who can write the service specification. Specifications are a form of technical writing when part of a contract, so getting this right is important. For a smaller specifications, a commissioning lead may write the specification and only require a brief check from someone with contract skills.

Ideally, the person who puts pen to paper needs to be involved from the service design phase onwards. This ensures they understand what they are writing and all the nuances that can be important.

The format

Decide what sections to include in the specification (see Table 5.4), clearly label these sections, and then complete with the relevant information. It is helpful to retain a similar structure for all specifications with one provider, and indeed for all providers where you can. This makes comparison and consistency easier to manage.

The service aims and outcomes, and the service description, are the sections which require most detail. Expect these to hold most of the wording. For the service description, break down the information into clearly labelled components, with a clear and logical flow. Use tables or diagrams if helpful. If a point is a must, then using the term 'The Provider must' will provide that clarity.

Write with clear language and avoid jargon. Do not use acronyms unless clearly spelled out at the outset and routinely used by all the parties.

The details

As well as the details of the model, consider including details such as:

- hours of operation;
- methods of delivery, such as face to face or online;
- data systems or data collation and handling/security requirements;
- access for people with recognised avoidable inequalities;
- personalised care requirements, such as in personalised care and support plans;
- service user surveys and collection of patient feedback;
- environmental or climate requirements that are applicable.

Some of these details may be captured in other schedules of the contract and I would suggest avoiding duplication where possible. Perhaps a pointer to the detail in another schedule will give assurance that all key information is included.

Operational service factors

This section notes operational factors for consideration when designing services. These are often essential for ensuring operational success – the best service design in the world won't work if, for example, there isn't enough staff or supporting infrastructures in place to support good practice. The operational factors listed here are not exhaustive, and there are many more that may be applicable. However, the elements included here apply to many service designs.

Planning capacity and managing demand

As local needs have been identified and analysis completed, there is already a good estimate of how many people will need to use the service. This will be the estimated **demand**. The new service should therefore plan for this number of people. This ability to see and offer care or treatment to a certain number of people, will be a service's **capacity**.

Despite all the best data analyses, these two don't always match as they should. In many instances the demand is higher than capacity, which creates a waiting list of people. A waiting list is often unavoidable but waiting times need to be as short as possible, and waiting people need to be managed. For example, people should know how long they may wait and what to do if they need support in the waiting period. Waiting lists are not only frustrating (with potential harmful consequences) for patients, but they can also create poor working conditions for staff as they battle to 'catch up' or manage people who have been waiting a long time. That said, with today's financial struggles for health and social care, waiting times are inevitable and commissioners and providers are increasingly accepting this undesirable position.

Note that urgent care or same-day services are different, as there are no waiting 'lists' for urgent care, just waiting at home, in rooms, or corridors. These services need to be safely staffed with the right skills, flexing up and down when required.

When designing a service, it is important to try to match up the capacity with the demand as far as possible. Some tips include:

- Ensure all possible sources of referral are considered when estimating demand. Is there an opportunity for these to increase with a new service in place that is more accessible?
- Use any common understanding of how many people a particular clinician can see in a session, or how many procedures or tests can be completed in a day, to estimate capacity.
- For community-based or home-based services, consider access issues and travel times for both staff and patients.
- Factor in an estimate of how many people may fail to attend for their appointment or have to cancel – for example, people with exacerbating conditions may be more likely to not attend.
- Factor in what disturbances in the service may force cancellations – for example, staff annual leave in holiday periods, study leave, sickness, a surgeon responding to emergency demand.
- Identify any potential bottlenecks, such as a requirement for an X-ray before an appointment when there are stretched X-ray services. These can have great effect on patient flow if not tackled.
- Consider national guidance on maximum waiting times – are escalation procedures needed when a list gets too long?
- Include protocols for managing waiting lists, such as communication with patients and simple advice for them while they wait.
- If the match between capacity and demand is expected to fluctuate greatly, the financial model may need to reflect that to manage the risk for both commissioner and provider.

Integration of services

Integrated care involves delivery of care by two or more professions or organisations. This is usually a good approach, as outcomes and experiences are often improved when organisations collaborate. The integrated care systems support this way of working and integrated care is a key focus of the NHS Long Term Plan.

The benefits are many but primarily include the following:

- Plans are wrapped around the whole person and all their needs, including multiple morbidities, emotional health and wellbeing, and social and environmental needs.

- Exacerbation of a condition because of the effect of physical symptoms on a person's mental health, and vice versa, are managed better.
- Resources are saved and delays reduced through avoiding duplication – examples include single assessments, with patients only having to tell their story once.
- Seamless transfer of care between providers with patients informed about what to expect means fewer people get lost in the system.
- Shared care records between organisations with a single set of notes on a patient means all professionals can access and input to this.
- Integrated care is often closer to home, timely, and safe.
- There is better support for families, carers, and loved ones.

The extent and opportunities for integration will vary for each service design, but these opportunities can be identified and the approach made a priority to harness the benefits. This aspect of service design will likely mean more people around the table working to secure an effective design, and it may well mean it takes longer to come to a workable solution, but the benefits will make this worthwhile.

Here are some top tips:

- When designing a physical health service, talk to mental health commissioners and providers, and vice versa to identify mutual patient support opportunities.
- When commissioning social care services, involve healthcare, and vice versa. Joint commissioning may well need special arrangements to manage governance, risk, and costs, but don't let these be a barrier. Consider pooling budgets or resources to ease financial risk.
- There may be opportunities to integrate with education, housing, justice, leisure, and VCSE services.
- Look for opportunities for shared assessments or to reduce other areas of duplication.
- If it is a large-scale integration with a whole-system approach, then strong leadership must be in place to support liaison and collaboration across organisational boundaries.

Workforce planning

The workforce are those people who deliver services, and they include not only clinicians and other professionals but also roles such as managers, administration staff, porters, and so on. There may be an abundance of funding, but if the required staff can't be recruited to deliver the service, then it is all for nothing.

Build into the design process a plan for the workforce. This should be short term to ensure implementation and to introduce changes, but also consider the long term to ensure retention and recruitment won't be an issue in the future.

Things to consider when planning for workforce include:

- A diverse workforce has been shown to have multiple benefits for both the organisation and the people they care for. Ensure fair and transparent procedures are in place and that people with protected characteristics have equal opportunities for recruitment and development.
- Staff development and training is vital to ensure workforce have the knowledge, skills, and confidence to work effectively. Staff development plans are crucial and must be in place to meet the needs of the service and its staff.
- Increasingly, there are roles that are difficult to recruit for due to a lack of trained and available staff. In these instances, consider both:
  o forward planning to 'grow your own' workforce and create training and development opportunities to make your services future safe;
  o adding new roles – workforce supply has led to the development of new roles such as assistant practitioners, pharmacy support roles, and nursing associates, and these are designed to support highly qualified staff and may be an option to address gaps.
- Protocols and procedures may be needed to support integration. Data sharing agreements will ease the sharing of confidential patient records, and staff passports can help ease the work of some staff across organisational boundaries, such as where a specialist nurse is working in the community on outreach from an acute employer.

- Available financial resources will have significant bearing on the choices for workforce. It is this financial burden that has often prompted commissioners and providers to be innovative with staff skill mix, considering options that may not be the norm but still meet patient needs safely and effectively.
- Don't forget unpaid carers – these people provide untold support to the NHS and social care. Make sure they are assessed for their own needs, supported, informed, and, where applicable, trained in caring duties (see more on unpaid carers in Chapter 9).

Shared care records

Complete, accurate, and timely information about the people coming through any service is crucial. Patient care information is often shared with their general practitioner or other professionals, such as social care professionals, and when integrating any part of the service, or when there are expected transfers of care, then shared care records are very important. Having accessible records eases this process and improves information quality. Not sharing this information can affect overall system efficiency and have a negative impact on the person's care, safety, and experience, and their needs and personal preferences may not be known or understood by staff caring for them.

The shared care record brings together key information about a person, from all the different providers involved in their care and support, to create a single electronic view of key information. This allows those involved in planning and delivering care to access up-to-date health and care information safely and securely, so that they can provide better joined-up care as the person moves between different parts of the health and social care system. It also prevents the person from repeating their story and provides assurance that their needs and preferences will be understood and taken into account.

There are many benefits of shared care records. The following is adapted from NHS England (NHS England, 2024e).

The benefits for individuals are:

- safer, more coordinated services;
- reduction in time by avoiding the need to repeat medical or social care history;

- fewer repeats of tests, appointments, and admissions;
- preferences and needs observed (usually in a personalised care and support plan);
- improved experience and continuity of care (seamless experience when moving between organisations);
- improved confidence in services.

For health and care professionals, the benefits are:

- less time spent seeking information;
- delivery of safer and more personalised care;
- ability to work more collaboratively across organisational boundaries;
- improved patient transfer across services, including discharge planning;
- improved staff satisfaction.

For integrated care systems, the benefits are:

- support for more integrated ways of working across health and social care;
- cost saving through more effective ways of working;
- improved workforce experience;
- enhanced service delivery plans and care pathways;
- opportunities for data-driven identification of local health priorities.

Content of shared care records will vary, but they often contain several key information points:

- name, date of birth, and NHS number;
- address, contact numbers, next of kin;
- allergies;
- diagnosis of any long-term conditions;
- test results;
- clinical care plans;
- personalised care and support plans, including personal preferences;
- discharge letters and care advice;
- appointments;

- inpatient stays;
- clinical contacts.

However, sharing information securely and having compatible IT systems is a book all on its own. The difficulties and barriers are well recognised, but if there is opportunity to develop shared care records, then it will be of enormous benefit. And there is increasing focus in NHS England on supporting this approach.

If you are seeking to implement or widen use of good shared patient record arrangements, then 'good' looks like:

- shared care records implemented across the locality for all relevant organisations;
- use of a consistent information standard so everyone is using the same terms and language;
- provision of real-time information to support effective management of patients;
- system capabilities for data sharing and easy sign-in authentication, compatible with digital disease plans;
- can be viewed by the patient or a person they nominate.

Good to know: Procurement rules

A lot of the work for service design is conducted alongside partners, and ideally it is co-produced. However, things become a little muddier when you are going out to procurement for a service. Here the procurement rules will come into play, you must tread carefully so you do not break rules around fair competition.

For example, if you work closely with a provider to design and then write a service specification, they will have a much greater advantage when it comes to bidding for the service when it goes out to tender. You and your organisation could be challenged on that. Where there are many potential providers who could bid on your procurement, then you must ensure fairness.

There were new rules introduced with the Health and Care Act 2022. From 1 January 2024, the Provider Selection Regime came into force. Now, where the provider in question is clearly the only provider who can deliver the services as required, the award of the contract can be made to them without a competitive process. In these instances, if you have reasonable grounds to believe they are the only suitable provider, then you can avoid the competitive process and the cost and resources burden this can carry. This approach aims to support the arrangement of services in the best interests of patients, taxpayers, and the population.

But if that is not the case, and you need, or there are clear benefits for, a full procurement, be careful in the process of writing the specification. Still involve your key partners and co-produce an approach, but keep the writing of the service specification within the commissioning body only. Open market testing can offer opportunities for providers to give feedback on the feasibility of your plans, and this approach will limit conflict of interest challenges which might apply if you only engage with one provider that is likely to be an interested party. Market testing through official channels allows you to share your potential model and invite in valuable provider views.

You can offer an 'input'- or 'output'-style service specification. For either choice, the bidding providers will need to have all the required information to offer a cost for the tender of that service or to decide if that it is possible to deliver the service within the specific budget you have set.

Procurement rules change from time to time, and these can have a big effect so always check the latest guidance for each new procurement. (See more on the NHS Provider Selection Regime at: www.england.nhs.uk/commis sioning/how-commissioning-is-changing/nhs-provider-selection-regime/)

REFLECTIONS FOR LEADERS

Leading change

Leaders in health and social care play an important part in enabling change. Change will often meet resistance, which can be due to many factors, such as traditional beliefs and practices, financial worry, or threat to jobs. The role of leaders is to facilitate the improvement and sustainability of the integrated care systems, and influencing and persuading partners to collaborate and cooperate is a leadership skill. It is leaders who oversee and facilitate the attainment of shared value-based goals while maintaining financial stability. Occasionally, difficult decisions will need to be made, such as whether to stop or dramatically change services. The rationale of these decisions needs to be clear and must be supported by the appropriate board(s) so that transparency of the decision-making process is beyond dispute.

Leaders need to take care that bureaucracy is not a barrier to change. Commissioners can sometimes be inflexible and resistant to change, especially when mindful of the potential risks and the use of taxpayer money. I would urge leaders to be open to change and innovation, especially as they stretch to reach the goals of a holistic model of health and wellbeing. For example, use outcome specifications to empower clinicians and providers or test new ways of working.

Another potential barrier is over-rigid strategy. Very detailed plans can often be beset with problems and then do not come to fruition. To overcome this, maintain flexibility in your strategy. Use your analysis to ensure you are addressing the right issues for the right people, but make the process of design incremental and emergent. Senior leaders can set broad goals and then trust those closer to the detail to implement effective change. This is a 'bottom-up' approach rather than a very planned 'top-down' process. It takes some confidence and trust. Putting into place some effective governance practices can provide appropriate assurance without them being a barrier.

Suggestions for success

Service design is part of the continuous cycle of improvement – however, always be aware of the upheaval and impact of change. Don't initiate change unless there is a clear sense of purpose and benefit. Staff can become change fatigued and demotivated if there is no stability period.

Don't underestimate the value of the vision and the importance of values – keep bringing what you are doing back to 'why'. Remember you are designing and implementing change for improvements to the lives of people, so keep this forefront.

6

Contracts

Aim

Contracts are the key vehicle for enabling and assuring effective changes made through commissioning. They document all the decisions and actions between partners and supports them with the backing of good governance. Understanding the contract, and using it to maximum benefit, is a key skill for commissioners. As well as the NHS standard contract, the use of other contracting models, such as those used in primary care and grants used with the voluntary, community and social enterprise (VCSE) sector, is covered.

The NHS standard contract

The aim of the contract

The NHS standard contract is a binding agreement between two or more parties – the commissioner and the provider – and it is mandated by NHS England. This formal approach helps commissioners ensure that providers comply with rules, regulations, and any local agreements. It protects all parties, as it is a formal record of what has been agreed and provides structure if difficulties arise.

The contract is mandated for use for all healthcare services (with some exceptions, covered in later in the chapter).

The contract is made up of three components and a fourth document is the technical guidance. The components are shown in Table 6.1.

Table 6.1: Components of the NHS standard contract

The component	What it is	Use
The particulars	The contract to which all the details agreed will be added. It contains the key schedules for completion and the signature page for signing by all parties.	This is the **key document**. This is the document that you will amend to meet your local arrangements, and it is this that you and the provider will sign and refer to for subsequent contract monitoring.
Service conditions	These are conditions relevant to service delivery. Not all conditions will be applicable for every arrangement – for example, ambulance requirements won't be needed for a mental health provider.	This is for information only and does not need to be exchanged between parties. It is applied automatically. It is mandated and cannot be amended.
General conditions	This sets out more general terms and conditions that are not applicable to services – for example, how the contract is managed.	This is for information only and does not need to be exchanged between parties. It is applied automatically. It is mandated and cannot be amended.
Technical guidance	This is the current guidance for each year's contract and sets out how to use the schedules.	This should be read thoroughly by commissioners each year. I would recommend a detailed read for each version, highlighting all the key changes and important actions.

The policy aim of the standard contract is not simply to allocate resources to providers; it is an instrument to improve services. It includes schedules that promote and support discussions and actions for improvement. The contract frequently includes changes to support and steer commissioners with national priorities – for example, schedule 2M was introduced in 2019 to support contracting discussions about personalised care.

Parties using the NHS standard contract

Providers

The contract should be used for all providers of services commissioned, regardless of service value or length of duration (so that includes pilots). There are a few exceptions, and these are:

- primary care, where the primary care contract should be used;
- financial support to VCSE organisations, where a grant agreement can be used;
- subcontracts from a provider to another provider – they will have to use alternative agreements.

There are two forms of the NHS standard contract. The **full-length** is the standard contract with all requirements included. Where a lighter touch is appropriate, the **shorter-form** contract can be used, such as when a small organisation is delivering only one service – for example, a hospice, a care home, or a pharmacy. The shorter-form contract restricts the detailed requirements and so is not appropriate for use with larger organisations or for services such as Accident and Emergency or inpatient services.

Commissioners

The commissioners using the NHS standard contract are typically integrated care boards and/or NHS England. Local authorities can use the contract, but they are not mandated to do so.

The contract can be both bilateral and multilateral. That means it can be used by a single commissioner or a group of commissioners who collaborate. Where this group approach is implemented, there is a nominated 'co-ordinating commissioner' who leads on behalf of the group.

There are benefits to working within a collaboration of commissioners. It promotes:

- a consistent approach across a patch;
- efficiency for both commissioners and providers due to only having to agree one contract and report to one team;
- increased likelihood of good practice being identified and implemented.

In a commissioner collaboration, a collaborative commissioning agreement is recommended. This document sets out how the arrangement will operate and how the commissioners will work together effectively. This agreement is not added to the contract, but the roles and responsibilities can be added to schedule 5C. Commissioner roles and responsibilities.

Completing the schedules

The schedules in the particulars are sections in the contract which group information together in categories. They are colour-coded in the contract. Red sections are mandatory and must not be altered or removed. Amber means for completion with local determination, but the sections must be completed. Green means optional and can be left blank if both parties agree to do so. For clarity, I would suggest rather than leaving any greens blank, you enter 'not applicable'.

Table 6.2 provides a summary of the schedules for the full-length contract. For an up-to-date explanation, always refer to the latest technical guidance, as there are updates every year.

Good practice tips:

- Delete any guidance notes that are included in italics – this will make the final document easier to read.
- Don't embed any documents in the contract. Instead enter the text in full in the appropriate section or reference the document title and then attach it to the contract as a sperate document.
- The NHS England NHS Standard Contract team offer help via email, which I recommend. They are usually quick to respond and very helpful. Also, get yourself on their mailing lists. Most years, they offer webinars or training sessions to explain any key changes from subsequent years. You can also be included in consultation on the planned changes for the next contract iterations.

Table 6.2: NHS standard contract schedules

Section	Status*	Purpose
Front page 1 and 2	A	Give a reference number or name to the contract and add essential details such as the date of agreement and the names of the key parties involved.
Signature page	A	The signature pages must be completed and shared between parties to make the contract legal and binding.
Service commencement and contract term	A	Add the dates of the contract agreement and when the service starts. A long stop date can be used for specifying a date when all outstanding arrangements must be fully in place. This date will be after the contract start date. Include how long the contract will last for and any potential extension periods agreed. Finally, add the notice periods required of both the commissioner and provider for full or part termination.
Services	A	List the services to which the contract is applicable. You can reference the prior approval timescales here if they apply.
Governance and regulatory	A	Add the names of key people for governance and regulatory duties. These named people will hold responsibility for important duties, such as safeguarding.
Contract management	A	Include the formal leads for contracting purposes, such as who to serve notice to. Include the frequency of contract review meetings and who the representatives from each party will be.

Schedule 1. Service commencement

A. Conditions precedent	A	This section sounds more complicated than it is – it covers everything that should be in place or defined before a provider can start a contract. That includes indemnity arrangements, CQC registration, and clarity on any subcontracting arrangements. There is a space to include other conditions precedent where applicable.
B. Commissioner documents	A	Share any documents the commissioner must make available to the provider before the contract starts – a local policy, for example.

Table 6.2: NHS standard contract schedules (continued)

Section	Status*	Purpose
C. Extension of contract term	A	This section is only to be used where, in a procurement exercise, a potential extension term has been advertised. Details are included here.
Schedule 2. The services		
A. Service specifications	A	Include all the agreed service specifications. If there is more than one specification, it is helpful to number them. There are sometimes specific specifications that must be used for certain services – for example, in 2023/24 there was a mandated specification for enhanced health in care homes and primary and community mental health services.
B. Indicative activity plan	A	Insert here any anticipated activity plans for each service, and if applicable, each commissioner. This will be an estimate of how many people or activity units (such as surgeries or X-rays) will be performed.
C. Activity planning assumptions	G	This space is for any assumptions used to calculate the indicative activity plan, such as: • external referral processes; • actions that the provider will employ to manage demand, such as first to follow up ratios; • assumptions used in estimates, such as numbers of emergency readmissions.
D. Essential services E. Essential services continuity plan	G	For NHS trusts, list here any essential services that must be provided – for example, Accident and Emergency services. Where this is appliable, a continuity plan must be in place and the title should be inserted here and the document attached to the final contract.
F. Clinical networks	A	If there are any applicable clinical networks that the provider must participate in, then list them here.
G. Other local agreements, policies, and procedures	A	Bit of a catch-all section – any policies or procedures that you want your provider to adhere to must be included here with the details. Prior approval schemes could be included.
H. Transitions arrangements	A	This won't be used often but sometimes where a new service is being introduced and it replaces another, the old provider will have to complete a series of actions to hand over control to the new provider.

(continued)

Table 6.2: NHS standard contract schedules (continued)

Section	Status*	Purpose
		This might include actions for staff, equipment, premises, patient records.
I. Exit arrangements	A	If at the end of the designated contract period there are any special arrangements or payments agreed, enter them here.
J. Transfer of and discharge from care protocols	A	Set out the requirements and processes of transferring care for a patient from one care setting to another. As integration of care increases, and we continuously seek smoother and seamless transitions of care between providers, this section will become more important. Don't waste the opportunity to be clear on the expectations and protocols that will satisfy this requirement, while being proportionate to the size and capacity of the provider.
K. Safeguarding policies and Mental Capacity Act policies	A	The provider will have written safeguarding policies for children and/or adults, and a Mental Capacity Act policy. They should be referenced here and attached to the final contract.
L. Provisions applicable to primary care medical services	A	Only use this schedule where there are requirements for interface with primary care. It can be used to consider any provisions needed to make the contract compliant with the primary care contracts, if required. There is more help on this complexity in the technical guidance.
M. Development plan for personalised care	G	This is optional but I would strongly recommend it is used for all contracts. Set out how you intend to develop personalised care approaches with the provider for the contract term. Even if this is only simple actions, it is still a move in the right direction. Or you can insert a more ambitious phased plan to increase the personalised care offer and reap the benefits.
N. Health inequalities action plan	G	Again, this is optional, but I would recommend this is used for all contracts. Whether the actions are simple or more complex, all providers should be working to reduce avoidable health inequalities.
Schedule 3. Payment		
A. Aligned payment and incentive rules	A	Aligned payment is an essential block payment to a provider (though there are some elective activity exceptions – more on this in Chapter 7).

Table 6.2: NHS standard contract schedules (continued)

Section	Status*	Purpose
		This section must be completed for all NHS trusts. You can include specifics about advice and guidance arrangements too. Include the fixed payments details for each commissioner.
B. Locally agreed adjustments to NHS Payment Scheme unit prices	A	If you have agreed with the provider any adjustments to the NHS Payment Scheme, include the detail here, using the appropriate templates.
C. Local prices	A	Insert here any local prices agreed (those prices not included in the NHS Payment Scheme; if they are alterations from the NHS Payment Scheme, they go in Schedule B).
D. Expected annual contract values	A	Insert the expected annual contract values for each commissioner. This is the grand total of all the schedules above, which is split into 12 monthly payments. If payment is to be anything other than one twelfth per month, then include those details here.
E. Timing and amounts of payments in first and/or final contract year	A	Where the first or last year of the contract arrangements is not 1 April to 31 March, enter how the payments timing and amounts of payments will operate here.
F. Commissioning for Quality and Innovation	A	Include any relevant CQUIN indicators here. These may be national or local.

Schedule 4. Local quality requirements

Local quality requirements	G	If you agree any local quality requirements, include the details here. These will be in addition to nationally set quality requirements in the service conditions.

Schedule 5. Governance

A. Documents relied on	A	This is not a legally binding part of the contract, but it is a useful space to include any documents that agreements may have been based around or agreements on additional matters. Make sure these documents do not conflict with the service or general conditions.

(continued)

113

Table 6.2: NHS standard contract schedules (continued)

Section	Status*	Purpose
B. Providers material subcontracts	A	Insert details where providers are using subcontractors. A material subcontractor is one where, without them, the provider could not deliver the service in question.
C. Commissioner roles and responsibilities	A	The roles and responsibilities agreed in the collaborative commissioner agreement can be included here where applicable.
Schedule 6. Contract management, reporting, and information		
A. Reporting requirements	A	This will include what the provider must report against for the contract. You will need to pick out data requirements relevant to the contract – perhaps grey out those not applicable. There is space at the end for local requirements.
B. Data quality improvement plans	A	If the data required for 'A. Reporting requirements' is not available or is not good quality, you may agree to improve the data in the data quality improvement plan. Use clear timescales and objectives.
C. Service development and improvement plans	A	This is a plan agreed with the provider, setting out the activities required to improve services commissioned. This is a useful mechanism to agree phased implementation of development to an existing service, or jointly tackle important priorities. You can use multiple service development and improvement plans where applicable.
D. Surveys	A	Insert any survey requirements, including national requirements and local agreements. Patient and staff surveys are usually the norm. You may wish to include details of specific content, timing, or frequency.
Schedule 6E. Data processing services		
Data processing services	A	This section is used as a data processing agreement. The provider is acting as a data processor – that is, they process (obtain, record, and hold) personal data on behalf of the commissioner. The table can be completed with the relevant details.
Schedule 7. Pensions		
Pensions	G	This is only used where staff have transferred over from another provider and pension rights need to be considered. I would suggest legal advice is sought before using this section.

Note: * R is for red – mandatory; A is for amber – for completion with local determination, but the sections must be completed; G is for green – optional and can be left blank.

Good to know: Prior approval schemes

It is not uncommon today for commissioners to have prior approval schemes in place with their providers. These are essentially a policy with criteria for accessing certain treatments. The treatments in question are usually those where there is some uncertainty about clinical value for some people. For example, a common procedure included in a prior approval scheme is tonsillectomy. The policy may state that a tonsillectomy should only be performed where the person in question has fulfilled the criteria, such as a minimum number of infections, or where there have been other clinical complexities. The rationale would be that the benefits of surgery for people who have had very few infections does not balance with the risks and costs of surgery. This approach can apply to many procedures. Some procedures will simply be 'not routinely funded' – that is, there is no criteria, as the commissioner does not see clinical value in any circumstance. Cosmetic procedures often fit into this category.

The prior approval policy can be shared with professionals at different stages of the patient's pathway – for example with the general practitioner (GP) or physiotherapist. But in some cases, the treatment is not decided until the person has seen a specialist consultant. Therefore, the prior approval processes need to be understood and practised at many tiers, but more so in the acute setting where the procedures take place most frequently. This can be an administrative burden, and this must be considered by commissioners as they develop their policy.

If a clinician finds that a person doesn't meet the prior approval criteria but does have some specific circumstances that make them clinically exceptional from other people, then they can apply to their commissioners through an individual funding request process. There will be a process in each integrated care system to deal with these requests. Typically, individual funding request panel members will meet frequently to consider each request on a case-by-case basis. Where there is true exceptionality, they will agree to fund the treatment in question without setting any precedent.

Managing the contract

Contracting monitoring

All contracts need to be managed well. This entails regular review of performance to provide assurance that all is working effectively, to ensure early identification of problems, and to maintain good communication and relationships between commissioner and provider. It is usual practice to agree a regular contract monitoring meeting schedule with opportunities to meet and discuss progress, issues, and future planning. For larger contract arrangements, this is usually monthly. For smaller contracting arrangements, less frequent meetings, perhaps quarterly, may be agreed, with monthly reporting requirements for submission. It's about proportionality of time for both the commissioners and the providers.

Always aim to develop good working relationships with providers and remember they are your partners. Encourage an environment where innovation and service improvements are welcomed and supported. Duty of candour (a legal responsibility to be open when things go wrong) is supported through non-judgemental conversations about mistakes made and the learning opportunities. Risks should be managed together, and it is sensible to have contingency plans in place in case problems develop. Ask providers to contribute to local needs assessments, and together start planning for future commissioning well ahead of the end of the contract.

A usual contract meeting will include (but is not limited to):

- discussion of submitted reporting on contract performance and quality indicators;
- consideration of any progress against schedules or development plans, such as the data quality and improvement plan or the service development and improvement plan;
- opportunity for the provider to share any incidents or identified risks;
- sharing of completed or in-progress quality improvement initiatives by the provider. This may be a result of quality audits or part of ongoing improvement programmes, not necessarily part of the contract agreement;
- opportunity for the commissioner or provider to share any relevant information, such as publication of refreshed standards, policies, or national plans;

- discussion of any payment or financial issues;
- discussion and agreement of any contract variations which may be applicable.

Contract variation

A contract variation is a tool for modifying an existing contract. They can be used when either:

- a multi-year contract is extending into the next financial year; or
- a mid-year change in contract is required.

There is a template available for commissioners and providers to use, and this is updated frequently. The most up-to-date version must be used in each case.

National variation

A national variation is a 'must-do' if applicable to your contract and provider. These are mandated changes that have been introduced by NHS England. They can introduce changes to the contract particulars, service conditions, or general conditions. Commissioners and providers must apply these variations as provided. If it is a significant change, then NHS England will usually suggest a reasonable time period within which to enact the changes.

Local variation

These are changes which have been locally agreed between the commissioner and provider, usually mid-year. A template is available to capture what has changed, and this includes a section for the new signatures.

An example of a local variation may be the agreement to implement a new service specification with a service change. In this example, the variation agreement may include the new specification (and specify what it replaces, if applicable) and any relevant inclusions to schedules, such as new reporting arrangements or additions to the data quality and improvement plan.

Levers and incentives

There are some levers and incentives that can be used by commissioners – a bit like a carrot and stick. The levers are the stick! I touch on these briefly and they can be useful at times, but I would use levers with caution. Nothing can replace good relationships with your partners, in which you support each other to achieve improved outcomes for patients. However, occasionally, you will need some help to manage a contract when there is lack of cooperation.

Contract levers

Financial sanctions

In my many years as a commissioner, I very rarely used the contractual levers to withhold money. My commissioning teams have always negotiated our way out of difficulties. I have infrequently used a **contract performance notice** to highlight the seriousness of an issue, but I would rarely apply financial sanctions as a coordinating commissioner. Use these with caution, as they can lead to further deterioration of performance when a provider is struggling financially, and they can damage trust and relationships. Use them as a last resort in a reasonable and proportionate way.

Good to know: Contract performance notice

A contract performance notice is issued by the commissioner when a provider has failed or is failing to comply with any of its obligations and the usual contract meeting discussions are not resolving the issue. The notice will signify the need for a contract management meeting. This is a one-off meeting to agree and implement a remedial action plan to get things going in the right direction. This plan may include actions for the provider alone or for the provider and commissioner. The plan sets out actions required to remedy the position and to specify what needs to happen for the provider to meet its contractual obligations. Specific and achievable actions are accompanied by realistic timeframes.

Financial sanctions, or withholding funds, play a lesser part in the current NHS standard contract nowadays, as it is increasingly recognised that they can do more harm than good. Sanctions are the financial consequences applied to providers for not upholding their contractual commitments. Examples where withholding sums can apply include the following (but always check the most recent contract rules):

- information breaches, where a provider has breached data security and has accidentally or unlawfully destroyed, lost, altered, disclosed, or accessed sensitive information;
- locally agreed consequences for failing to meet a quality requirement that is important;
- failure of the provider to attend a contract management meeting following a contract performance notice, or if they will not agree a remedial action plan;
- force majeure, which refers to the very rare occasions where events or circumstances out of the parties' control makes the provider unable to comply with the terms – this could be a flood, terrorism, or riots.

In the examples here, sums are generally withheld until a plan of rectification, usually the remedial action plan, has been agreed and implemented. Payment can then resume.

Inspection and assurance

This is a reputational and quality lever that promotes the provision of quality services. The Care Quality Commission (CQC) regularly assesses sites delivering NHS services to ensure they provide high-quality, safe, and effective services to patients. This includes hospitals, GP surgeries, care homes, and others. Services are measured against a set of national standards, and results are published for everyone to access. Most hospitals, care homes, and domiciliary care services are inspected at least once a year.

There are requirements in the NHS standard contract that align with CQC standards – for example patient safety in the service conditions. Commissioners have the option to report any non-compliance to the CQC. The CQC then has power to enforce improvements, fine providers for breaches, and stop any unsafe practice.

Good to know: Care Quality Commission

The Care Quality Commission, more commonly referred to as the CQC, is an independent body that regulate health and social care in England. It is their responsibility to ensure that care is safe, effective, high quality, and compassionate. All providers for health and social care must have CQC registration to operate. This includes services for treatment of a disease, disorder, or injury; diagnostic and screening procedures; personal care services; accommodation for care; supply of blood products; medical transport services; and maternity and midwifery services. The five questions asked of these providers (see CQC, 2022) are:

- Are they safe?
- Are they effective?
- Are they caring?
- Are they responsive to people's needs?
- Are they well led?

This well-balanced mix is an assuring method of regulating provider quality.

The CQC key duties include the monitoring of all providers (NHS and non-NHS providers) who require registration. This is predominantly conducted via inspections of providers. Where there is a failing in standards, the CQC can take steps to ensure improvements are made. These can include changing a provider's registration, and therefore how they can operate, putting a provider in 'special measures' with close supervision until improvements are made, or issuing cautions, fines, and even prosecuting where there are serious failings.

In 2023 the testing phase of inspections for integrated care systems began. We can expect to see a new model of inspections developed for system leaders in the near future.

Contract incentives

Commissioning for Quality and Innovation framework

The Commissioning for Quality and Innovation (CQUIN) payment framework enables commissioners to reward providers for delivering specific quality and innovation improvement goals, which are selected nationally each year, for maximum benefit, by NHS England. The goals link a proportion of the providers' income to their achievement. This is a small proportion and in 2023/24 it was only 1.25 per cent of the fixed income value. Currently, this scheme is only applicable to contracts above £10 million on the full-length NHS standard contract. CQUIN goals appear in the particulars section of the contract under the national and local quality requirements.

In addition to the national CQUIN goals, or for those contracts where the national scheme does not apply, commissioners can agree local CQUIN goals or an equivalent. Should you use local CQUIN goals? Some recent reviews have concluded that the evidence of the impact of CQUIN goals on outcomes is limited, and the non-recurrent funding arrangement does not allow recurrent investment in the service. However, careful construction of CQUIN goals alongside regular assessment of progress may increase the potential for impact. Allowing the incentive to remain in place over a longer period to encourage greater planning is beneficial, where it is possible to do so.

If you do decide to agree local CQUIN goals, the design will require, as a minimum:

- a clear standard to reach or improve on – be specific;
- a means of measuring progress from the current position to the ideal future position – there needs to be enough data in place currently to set a baseline position;
- an exit strategy (to normalise the improvement once reached, so that CQUIN payment can cease).

Best practice tariffs

Best practice tariffs are a part of the NHS Payment Scheme (discussed in Chapter 7). These are formal prices applied to defined quality-based activities or those that are cost-effective. They have been around since 2010 but are updated at intervals.

As these tariffs are generous, they incentivise a shift from usual care to that which is best practice. They are individual in their remit but they tend to share characteristics, such as:

- reducing avoidable admissions;
- delivering care in appropriate settings;
- promoting quality accreditation of providers (formal confirmation of quality provision);
- improving quality of care.

Although best practice tariffs may appear costly to commissioners, they should be viewed as 'invest to save' initiatives. That is, they will not only improve outcomes and experiences for people, but also save the system costs of unnecessary admissions, or exacerbation of conditions leading to future care costs.

Informal incentives

There are a range of informal incentive approaches that commissioners can use to promote the safe and effective delivery of services. The following may be useful to consider:

- providers affiliating with networks – these can be managed networks (usually funded with robust governance arrangements) and/or clinical networks (led by clinicians). These networks usually meet as an alliance of partners to examine how care in a particular care group can be improved. They can support identifying best practice, benchmarking, highlighting risks, and applying pressure on providers and commissioners where things are not going well. The reputational weight of performing well for networks is a great incentive. Commissioners can specify that the affiliation is enacted;
- providers working with communities and local voices – these are organised groups of people from local communities who can act as a voice for the population, providing insight into what works well and not so well. Maintaining good relationships with these groups is an incentive for providers to do well. Commissioners can specify how this will look in practice within their contracts;

- partnership working for the integrated care system, at place or neighbourhood level – within the NHS structures recently introduced, there is an increased focus on sustainability and joint working across organisations. This integrated approach of mutual benefit can be an incentive for providers to act with improvement in mind and with financial responsibility, so the wider area benefits from improved outcomes. Commissioners can ensure providers are connected and active using the most appropriate collaboration arrangement.

Contract length of term and decommissioning

Contract term

Many contracts will continue (with amendments) into the next contracting year, as it is too time consuming, expensive, and complex to do otherwise if performance is good. However, it is still good practice to share contracting intentions at an appropriate point to signal that it is the intent of the commissioners to continue the arrangement. Both parties can and should do this.

Where a service has gone through a formal procurement, there is often a determined period for the contract length – usually several years. The agreement cannot continue past the pre-agreed term, as this would breach procurement rules. Contract extension periods (usually one or two years) can be agreed in advance as part of the procurement process. At the end of the formal term, these extensions can be applied where both parties agree to do so. Anything exceeding these pre-agreed terms will usually need a new procurement or a clear rationale as to why a procurement is not needed.

Decommissioning

Decommissioning will not be needed often, but commissioners may need to consider exit strategies, decommissioning processes, and giving notice for the end of contract, if required.

If there is a need to end a contract, or a service within a contract, this will mean decommissioning. This need for decommissioning occasionally happens where there is no longer a clear service need, where the provider hasn't been working to the required standard, or where there is a new service to replace it. If a commissioner is ending a contract in full, then this is a **termination**.

In these scenarios, as much notice as possible should be given to the provider.

The contract gives some guidance on what should be considered for decommissioning and termination, and that includes arrangements for staff and other considerations. As decommissioning can have a very large impact, the approach must be robust and comprehensive, to minimise risk and disruption. The National Audit Office has a useful decommissioning toolkit for VCSE providers, but the principles are the same for most types of health and care provision (National Audit Office, nd).

The principles from the National Audit Office (2011) guide have been adapted and are shared next (notice that they mirror the commissioning cycle and are good commissioning principles in general):

1. Ensure good communication – maintain open, honest, regular, and transparent engagement and consultation with service providers.
2. Understand needs and the provider market – a good understanding of users' needs, the existing services that meet those needs, and the wider provider market will help when considering decommissioning options, risks, impacts, and effects on users and providers.
3. Focus on users and the community – a strong focus on users, not services, will help rationalise why a decommissioning decision has been made.
4. Have a clear rationale – consensus on the reasons why service change is needed can ensure key individuals and stakeholders 'own' the process and outcomes and can reduce mistrust from users and providers.
5. Understand impact – a robust process of impact analysis that looks at long-term 'whole life' impacts of services on users, providers, and the wider community can strengthen the case for change and offer better value for money.
6. Ensure robust risk management – identifying risks with the decommissioning process and to all stakeholders involved can make the process easier, reduce any fear or anxiety, and allow opportunity for mitigation.

7. Understand costs – having a clear understanding of what the current costs (and benefits and savings) of a service are and the potential future costs and benefits can help in assessing value for money.
8. Practise good governance – a clear decision-making process and governance structure will allow all stakeholders to understand roles and responsibilities and ensure a clear process for decommissioning.

Other contracting approaches

Primary care contracting

Primary care services include GP services, dentistry, opticians, and pharmacy. The way that primary care is contracted for is very different from other health services. In this section, I examine GP services, but be aware that there are different, though similar, arrangements in place for the other primary care services.

As from April 2023, the integrated care boards took delegated authority to discharge a range of NHS England statutory functions. This included delegated responsibility for commissioning primary care services. When integrated care boards assume responsibility for the delegated functions, they take on the liability for those functions, but in this case NHS England will retain overall accountability and therefore requires the necessary assurances that its functions are being discharged safely, effectively, and in line with the legal requirements. Assurance frameworks will support that process, with integrated care boards reporting to NHS England on this function.

Unlike many health service providers, GPs are small to medium businesses where the GP, or a partnership of GPs, share the income they generate. There are three contracts which can be used. These are:

- General Medical Services – this is the national standard contract and approximately 70 per cent of GP practices use this.
- Personal Medical Services – this is agreed locally and so has more flexibility than the General Medical Services contract. Around 26 per cent of practices use this form.
- Alternative Provider Medical Services – this contract offers the maximum flexibility. It can be used for provision of primary care services by independent providers other than GPs. This is in place for around 2 per cent of all the primary care contracts.

If a GP practice wanted to provide an NHS service that is not primary care, they would need to agree the arrangements in an NHS standard contract, just like any other provider.

Network Contract Direct Enhanced Service

An enhanced service is essentially a contract add-on. These can be direct, meaning they are nationally set, or local, meaning they are locally agreed. The Network Contract Direct Enhanced Service (DES) is a national requirement. It is a contractual vehicle to support primary care networks. It sets out the core requirements of a primary care network, but also what they are entitled to. For the DES, there was a financial commitment from NHS England of over £2 billion in 2023/24, with a proportion of the money earmarked for health professionals who can support delivery on the commitments. This includes, among other professionals, physiotherapists, pharmacists, and social prescribing link workers.

Included within the DES is the investment and impact fund. This fund is an investment scheme used to incentivise quality improvement and the achievement of the aims in the NHS Long Term Plan. The scheme contains indicators that focus on where primary care networks can contribute significantly towards the 'triple aim':

- improving health and saving lives;
- improving the quality of care for people with multiple morbidities;
- helping to make the NHS more sustainable.

Over £300 million was committed to this scheme in 2023/24, so it is a significant investment to support the development of the primary care networks. Each primary care network must reinvest this money into future service development and workforce.

Quality and Outcomes Framework

GP practices receive income for specified streams of activity, including core services and out-of-hours provision. I do not examine these in depth here, but it is useful to understand the Quality and Outcomes Framework (QOF), which works as an incentive scheme to reward work in priority areas. The QOF accounts for around 10 per cent of a practice's income. It is a voluntary programme that practices can opt in to. They receive payments based on good performance against several indicators. The framework covers a range of clinical areas – for example, management of hypertension or asthma; prescribing safety; and ill health prevention activity. Each area has a range of indicators that equate to a number of QOF points. At the end of the year, the practice receives a payment based on the points they have earned. Commissioners should understand this system because QOF indicators are a priority for practices, and they often spend a lot of time and effort in achieving their QOF points. Therefore, the practice can be a helpful partner in several ways, including developing pathways which are linked to QOF or providing good data on QOF populations. It is helpful for commissioners to be aware of what is in the QOF each year and to see what opportunities this may lead to for improving care.

Grant agreements

Grant agreements are the documentation used for less formal arrangements where a full legal contract is not required but commissioners would benefit from the details they have agreed being set down on paper for clarity of expectations. A grant is often used when commissioners are *supporting* a charity or VCSE sector service with funding. This is different from a contracting arrangement, where a commissioner is *purchasing* services.

There are templates for grants available on the NHS standard contract area (see: www.england.nhs.uk/nhs-standard-contract/grant-agreement/). These templates are a helpful starting point and can be adapted as required. My recommendation is to use the template and then in 'Schedule 1. The project', insert a mini service specification with key details of your expectations. 'Schedule 2. The grant' will include the details of the funding available and how and when it will be paid.

Grants are not subject to procurement rules, but when commissioners are awarding a large sum of money, it is good practice to be transparent about how, and why, the particular provider was chosen for the grant.

Social care frameworks

The continuing care arrangements are covered in Chapter 7 as a funding arrangement, and personal health budgets are discussed in Chapter 10. Here, I take a brief look at how local governments manage the contractual arrangements for providers of care services. This may be for homecare providers, supported living services, and residential or nursing care providers.

Due to the nature of the work, with it being unpredictable and changing for each client, providers tend to be asked to go through a procurement exercise to prove quality standards and legal requirements are in place. Those who are successful are then placed on a 'framework' list. They can be called on to accept or reject a call for services as and when a patient needs it.

Each local government will use identical framework agreements for each provider on the framework. For example, where a provider or several providers have won a tender for homecare services, they will all sign a contract with same terms and conditions and a service specification. The service specification will match the requirements of a particular social care service, also called 'lots'. Providers can apply to be on the framework for multiple lots. Because of the high numbers of people, the social care sector would not run effectively without private sector suppliers, and they make up most of the provision.

REFLECTIONS FOR LEADERS

Agreeing an effective contract

In my experience, most of the contractual detail is agreed between the commissioner and provider contracting teams. More senior leaders are required to facilitate discussions on tricky issues and to ensure that the bottom-line agreements are meeting strategic and financial aims.

Leaders should ensure that improvement is key within all contracts. One approach is to apply strategic aims to all contracts, making use of their structure and consistency. For example, the integrated care system will aim to agree change for implementing improvement in a priority area to all applicable providers. The trick is to not see the contract as just a formal bureaucratic requirement, but instead as an opportunity to promote and strengthen meaningful change.

Suggestions for success

The contract is necessary as a legal requirement; however, it can be contentious, and it can potentially drive barriers between you and your providers, affecting relationships that you may have worked hard to develop. Try to bear this in mind as you implement the contract, and be reasonable and fair. Preserve good working relationships as far as possible. Make joint decisions or explain those made as commissioners. Give opportunities to talk through issues, agreeing joint methods of action. Try to keep relationships positive and remind everybody of the shared vision to improve outcomes for people.

7

Funding approaches

Aim

This chapter demystifies the new NHS England funding models, improving understanding of how they work and why they are an aid to today's commissioning aims. This includes the blended payment approach but also other payment alternatives to support commissioning for outcomes. Limited funding or complicated finance arrangements are often regarded as one of the biggest barriers for commissioning and service redesign. This is because financial sustainability is a major risk and affordability is nearly always a factor. Because of this, the chapter also covers alternative funding approaches and ways to find the money.

History of NHS tariff schemes

Figure 7.1 shows the key changes in NHS funding approaches from 2003/04 to 2023/24. The NHS Payment Scheme was introduced in 2023/24 but aspects of the scheme had been slowly rolled out prior to this.

With a very brief look at NHS payment history, the tariff schemes – Payment by Results (2003/04 onwards) and the National Tariff (2014/15 to the introduction of the NHS Payment Scheme) – were used to set the rules and prices that commissioners needed to pay providers. These schemes were predominantly used for acute hospital care, and payment made from these schemes made up approximately 60 per cent of a hospital's income (NHS

Figure 7.1: Timeline of NHS funding models

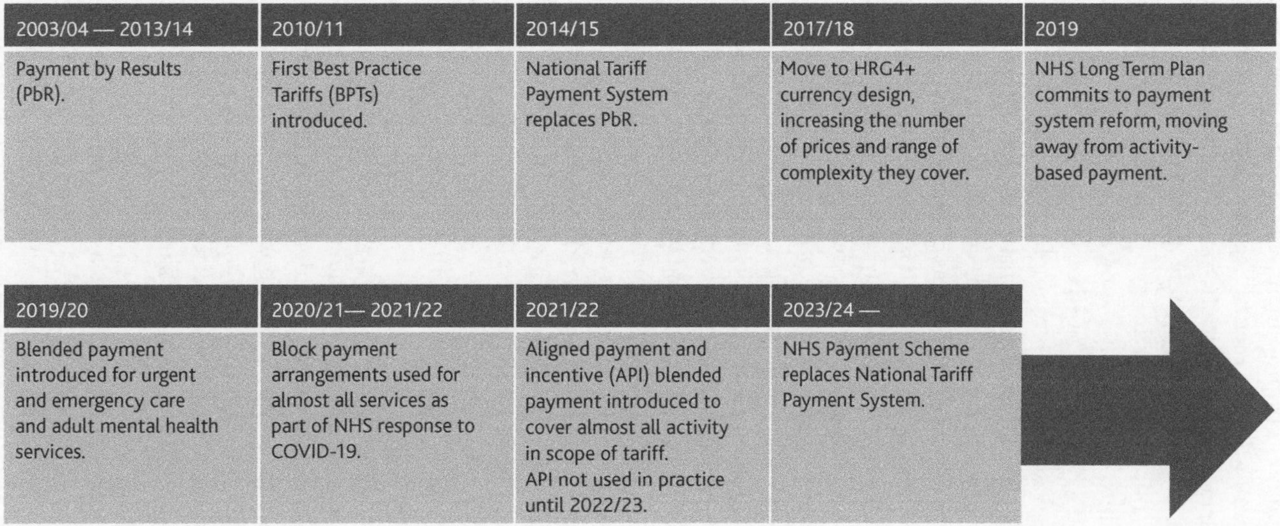

2003/04 — 2013/14	2010/11	2014/15	2017/18	2019
Payment by Results (PbR).	First Best Practice Tariffs (BPTs) introduced.	National Tariff Payment System replaces PbR.	Move to HRG4+ currency design, increasing the number of prices and range of complexity they cover.	NHS Long Term Plan commits to payment system reform, moving away from activity-based payment.

2019/20	2020/21 — 2021/22	2021/22	2023/24 —
Blended payment introduced for urgent and emergency care and adult mental health services.	Block payment arrangements used for almost all services as part of NHS response to COVID-19.	Aligned payment and incentive (API) blended payment introduced to cover almost all activity in scope of tariff. API not used in practice until 2022/23.	NHS Payment Scheme replaces National Tariff Payment System.

Source: NHS England (2023b) Open Government Licence v3.0

England and NHS Improvement, 2022a). Other service providers, such as community and mental health providers, remained largely on block arrangements, with no or few individual prices for units of activity. A block arrangement provides a set monetary value based on anticipated activity volumes and costs. This is usually then split into 12 monthly payments.

The tariff schemes were based on units of activity, to which a code and a price was applied. For example, a first outpatient appointment with a diabetes consultant would have a treatment function code 307 and attract a price of £137. This coding arrangement was applied for consultations, procedures, units of care, and investigations. It also reflected patient complexity – that is, how many conditions a person had, their age, how long they stayed in hospital, what professionals they saw, and so on. A single episode of care could have many codes. Coded activity translated into a price which commissioners were obliged to pay. Therefore, it was financially beneficial as a provider to get your coding completed thoroughly. The acute providers had teams of coders applying codes to all activity they completed. Professionals were trained in using the codes and the providers worked hard, using codes fully, to ensure no income was lost. Regarding data collection, this was great news. The availability and complexity of data going into acute care was excellent. However, there were risks and disincentives for all parties with the tariff approach.

For commissioners, these included:

- cost risk with acute care if demand into the hospital could not be controlled;
- costs spiralling as more people were identified as having more than one condition or several risk factors;
- lack of appetite from providers to develop integrated care pathways and coordinated approaches, as it would mean loss of income;
- reduced predictability of costs for acute care, as commissioners must pay for fluctuating demand.

For acute care providers, the risks and disincentives were:

- burden of coding all activity and the costs incurred;
- reduced predictability of costs with fluctuating demand;

- disincentive for acute providers to support alternative pathways of care for people elsewhere in the system, as this would mean loss of income (though in reality, many acute hospitals struggled with managing demand despite the funding it attracted);
- need for providers to manage services within national coding prices, which did not always match local costs;
- some potential to skimp on quality to see more patients and maximise profit.

For community and mental health providers, the risks and disincentives were:

- those who had block arrangements were more reluctant to accept additional referrals from acute care settings – they needed to balance the books within a set financial value, and if they saw more patients than anticipated, it was a risk to them financially and regarding the quality of care they could provide;
- the data from those with block arrangements was a lot poorer in quality and quantity, as there was no incentive to record the activity in such detail.

So, in summary, there were risks for all involved and disincentives for change, especially for integrated care models. In 2023/24, the NHS Payment Scheme was introduced with the aim of tackling these risks.

The NHS Payment Scheme

Funding flows

Under the new NHS structure, funding is cascaded down from the Department of Health and Social Care through NHS England, as shown in Figure 7.2. Here the funding is split into that required by integrated care systems and primary care, and as at 2023/24, some funding is separately allocated for specialised commissioning, but this will be delegated to integrated care systems in the future.

The integrated care systems will have responsibility for dividing available funding to the providers. Primary care, social care, and public health are outside of the NHS Payment Scheme.

Figure 7.2: Flow of NHS funding

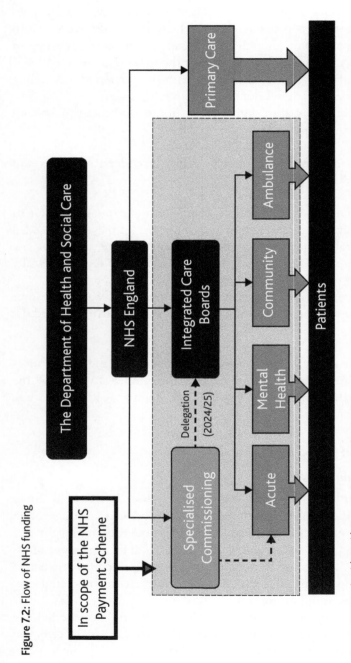

Enactment of the NHS Payment Scheme

The NHS Payment Scheme aims to achieve a more balanced approach to funding acute care provider contracts. One of the key components of the scheme is **blended payment**. Blended payment aims to take a blend of a **fixed element**, like the traditional block approach, and a **variable element**, like the old tariff approach. The combination of these two removes some of the old issues and maximises the benefits. In addition to these elements, the blended payment approach can include a **risk-sharing element** and/or a **quality- or outcomes-based element**. Table 7.1 summarised the elements of blended payment.

Table 7.1: Elements of blended payment

Element	Aim	Example
Fixed element	Value set based on forward-looking forecasts of activity and costs	A block payment that covers staff and running costs for the forecasted activity of a service where activity levels tend to be predictable.
Variable element	A predefined cost per unit	A tariff approach is applied for specific activity that is high cost or less predictable, for example complex operations or long-stay admissions. For 2023/24, these are the NHS Payment Scheme unit prices for elective activity.
AND OPTIONALLY		
Risk-sharing element	An agreement to share costs that fall above or below threshold limits, thereby sharing risk of under- or over-performance for less predictable activity	Thresholds (pre-agreed cut-off points) applied where reductions are made for less activity completed than planned or additional payments made for activity completed over and above the plan.
AND OPTIONALLY		
Quality or outcomes-based element	Incentive payments for completion of quality or outcomes-based goals	Percentage of contract value paid on completion of quality goals or outcomes achieved – for example increase in completed personalised care and support plans.

During 2023–25, the NHS Payment Scheme is to be enacted in four ways. These are:

- aligned payment and incentive approach – covers almost all NHS provider activity with fixed and variable elements;
- low-volume activity block payments – for provider arrangements worth less than £500,000;
- activity-based payments – for non-NHS providers delivering services with NHS Payment Scheme unit prices;
- local payment arrangements – locally agreed approaches where the above do not apply.

Aligned payment and incentive approach

The aligned payment and incentive approach is the key method in blended payment. Most NHS arrangements utilise this approach.

First, the blended payment fixed element value captures the estimated non-elective activity and the costs associated with the plan for the forthcoming year. This element considers the costs of an efficient provider, who strives for the best care and experience for patients. It needs to reflect certain assumptions about the volume of patients and their anticipated needs. It also includes an assumption that Commissioning for Quality and Innovation (CQUIN) targets will be met in full.

Second, a set price applies to all elective activity using the NHS Payment Scheme unit prices – this is the variable element. The provider is paid for the actual eligible activity they provide month on month. For acute providers; this is a very large amount of activity to be paid using unit prices, and this is contradictory to the initial aim of the scheme, which was to move away from the counting and coding limitations. For 2023–25, this approach of expanding the variable element to such a wide scope is referred to as the **Elective Recovery Fund**. This approach incentivises providers to clear the post-pandemic backlog. This part of the aligned payment and incentive approach will largely affect acute providers. Community and mental health providers will have a larger fixed element, with very little or no elective unit prices applicable.

Low-volume activity

Low volume activity arrangements are applied where a contract value is not expected to exceed £500,000. These arrangements support effective flows of payment between commissioner and provider without being burdensome. This covers acute, community, and mental health services with a few specific exceptions, such as inpatient out-of-area placements. This refers to small provider arrangements that are usually outside of the geographical area, such as students cared for in university towns or people treated while on holiday.

NHS England have a schedule of each of these arrangements for all commissioners. Using a three-year rolling average, a sum is set nationally for commissioners to pay each year. There would be no other transactions in-year.

Activity-based payments

If a non-NHS provider is providing elective activity which has a NHS Payment Scheme unit price, then an activity-based mechanism applies and the nationally set prices will be used. This is commonly the case for independent providers offering certain surgeries, such as orthopaedic procedures, where the local acute providers are struggling with demand.

In these cases, there is likely to be very little or no fixed element.

The best practice tariff will apply where providers have achieved the specified standards for each tariff, as will specialised services top-ups where the services in scope are provided (see Table 7.2).

Local payment arrangements

There is scope to apply a locally designed blended payment model to other commissioning arrangements where they do not fit into the categories mentioned earlier or where there are circumstances that warrant a change. Circumstances where a local arrangement may be applied include:

- funding of service development improvements and service transformation;
- funding of initiatives to address health inequalities;
- where historic efficiencies have been achieved that will affect prices – for example, where service redesign has shown savings with lower indicative costs than the NHS Payment Scheme unit prices;
- where there are differences in costs incurred by different types of providers and in different areas (sometimes using benchmarking).

Table 7.2: NHS Payment Scheme terms

High-cost exclusions	These items and activity are excluded from the general scheme because they are specialist or bespoke and costs can vary dramatically. It would be difficult to determine a fair set price for these, because how and when they are used is so different across the country. Therefore, it is fairer to exclude them and allow local negotiations to confirm an arrangement. These include: • high-costs drugs; • high-cost devices; • MedTech Funding Mandate products – selected innovative medical devices and digital products which the NHS Long Term Plan is supporting accelerated rollout for; they are NICE recommended, and they meet the criteria to save costs and resources and make a return on investment within three years; • homecare services providing care in the patient's own home. These are excluded from the aligned payment and incentive approach and arrangements for paying for these need to be agreed locally.
Commissioning for Quality and Innovation	As of 2023/24, the CQUIN value is set at 1.25% (NHS England, 2023f) but this can vary year on year. For NHS Payment Scheme, the CQUIN is assumed achieved as part of the fixed element, and adjustments are made at year end if this is not the case. In most cases, it is easy for commissioners and providers to identify relevant CQUIN goals and to slot them into the contract. Those that do not apply are ignored. Commissioners can choose alternatives to the nationally set CQUIN goals for contracts with a value of less than £10 million. This is to ensure that the CQUIN framework remains meaningful and effective for all circumstances. CQUIN is discussed as an incentive in Chapter 6.

Table 7.2: NHS Payment Scheme terms (continued)

Best practice tariffs	Best practice tariffs are a unit price designed to incentivise quality and cost-effective care. For the NHS Payment Scheme, the best practice tariffs scheme in 2023–25 is split into an annual achievement value that is bundled into the fixed element. Where it applies to elective activity, the costs will be part of the variable element for the aligned payment and incentive approach. (Best practice tariffs are discussed as part of the contract in Chapter 6.)
Prescribed specialist service top-ups	Prescribed specialist services are those identified for joint commissioning between integrated care boards and NHS England. This arrangement was launched in 2023 with greater statutory responsibility by the boards from 2024 onwards. Identification rules help commissioners identify those services which are classed as prescribed specialist services, as this can be quite complex. These services will attract a top-up payment to reflect the costs of delivery. For the NHS Payment Scheme, prescribed specialist services is paid as part of the variable element, rather than on a fixed basis. The top-ups are added to the unit prices where they apply. Integrated care boards participating in this delegated arrangement will receive an allocation to reflect these extra costs.
Market factor forces	Market factor forces attempt to estimate the unavoidable cost differences between healthcare providers. These could include the rurality of an area, costs of land or buildings, and staffing costs. Market factor forces aims ensure that providers and their patients are not advantaged or disadvantaged by these cost differences. Each provider has a market factor forces rating or index value based on their location. The integrated care system allocations are then adjusted so that they can afford to pay for the same level of care wherever they are in the country.
Cost uplift and efficiency factor	These are annual adjustments made nationally that account for inflation costs (an uplift) and annual efficiency savings (a decrease). The combination of the two gives a final percentage uplift or decrease. The inflation costs consider inflation and forward-looking costs, such as staff pay awards, costs of drugs, capital costs, energy costs, and fuel. The efficiency factor is an average estimate of what is achievable for providers. There is constant pressure to do more with less.

Where integrated care boards wish to apply local variations to the aligned payment and incentive approach and the unit prices, they need to seek approval from the regional NHS England teams. The regional teams recognise that localities have varying needs and that there will be a need in some areas to do something different.

Applying the NHS Payment Scheme terms

The NHS Payment Scheme, particularly the aligned payment and incentive approach, have terms and conditions, and uplifts and decreases are applied, which vary from place to place and from contract to contract. There are a number of arrangements with specific terms applied to them. Table 7.2 sets out the key terms to be aware of.

Good to know: Key terms for contractual activity

Elective: Planned activity that is not urgent – for example, a referral to see a consultant or a planned surgery.

Non-elective: Unplanned activity that is urgent or an emergency – for example, Accident and Emergency attendances or overnight stays for urgent clinical need.

Out-patient: A meeting (face to face, virtual, or by telephone) with a professional to discuss symptoms or a condition. This can include tests, care, or treatments.

Inpatient: An admittance to a ward for an overnight stay. This can be for care, treatment, or investigations.

Follow-up: A further meeting after a first outpatient appointment or an admittance. This is to review symptoms or condition and see if further action or advice is required.

Day case: These are procedures undertaken on one day with no need for an overnight stay. The patient is sent home on the same day as the procedure.

Payment schemes for commissioning priorities

The NHS Payment Scheme is evolving, and it aims to meet the needs of the system at any given time. For example, the 2023–25 scheme aims to support the recovery of the impact left by the global pandemic. Waiting lists, with impacts on patients' health and wellbeing, are high so the scheme uses the key components of the approach but in a bespoke way that benefits the whole system. For this period, the scheme prioritises the payment of elective (planned) activity with fair prices to help providers reduce waiting lists and see people as quickly as possible. The NHS Payment Scheme will alter again from 2025 onwards to meet new priorities, but it will continue to apply the same aims of (adapted from NHS England, 2023b):

- application in the best interests of patients, such as supporting quality, cost effectiveness, innovation, and managing risk;
- promotion of transparency and good data quality to improve accountability and encourage sharing of best practice;
- constructive engagement between commissioner and provider, including the relationships with clinicians, patient groups, and other relevant stakeholders;
- contribution to reducing health inequalities – for example, providing equitable access, good experiences for all, and optimum outcomes for population cohorts;
- delivering the aims of the operational planning guidance.

The NHS Payment Scheme and its application are complex. There are many rules and considerations for applying the scheme. This book does not attempt to replicate the guidance that is provided year on year to help commissioners and providers through the process. However, the blended payment approach looks here to stay, and it is important to understand how it works in practice.

Good to know: Operational planning guidance

Every year, usually in December, NHS England shares the priorities for the year ahead through operational planning guidance. This guidance aims to set out what the national objectives are and what integrated care systems will be expected to do to help achieve this. This guidance also sets out how NHS England assesses performance against these priorities.

This guidance is always waited for with anticipation, as it steers the strategic planning and contractual agreements for the coming year. There is the added complexity of seeing how these national objectives fit with the local priorities already identified and aimed for.

Applying blended payment to other providers

The NHS Payment Scheme is for acute care predominantly, so how can blended payment be applied to other sectors, such as community services or mental health? Table 7.3 provides examples of how the blended model can be applied for different providers.

Good to know: Open book accounting

Open book accounting is the process of openness and transparency between commissioner and provider on their financial positions. It builds trust, as it demonstrates there is no profiteering or inflated charging by the provider. Plus, because the commissioner can see where a trust or organisation is struggling financially, they may be more able to work together towards sustainable solutions.

The sharing of accounts facilitates honest public debate about the costs of care and the impact of future initiatives or funding models. It is a pain/gain share whereby both parties own the costs and the burden of financial stability.

This is a big cultural change for many, and communication and trust are as important to the success of this approach as systems and processes are.

Table 7.3: Application of blended payment for providers in different sectors

Sector	Blended payment arrangement
Community	Most of this arrangement will be a fixed element. This will be based on previous volumes with any assumptions about future activity flows applied – for example, a new service pathway. A local arrangement can be applied to add a variable element, which could be linked to less predictable activity or can be used to apply community currency activity. A further element can be linked to quality initiatives – for example, payment linked to supported self-management programme participants, or those accessing a new service transformation model. Risk shares are optional but could be applied if there is any activity that is unpredictable but resource heavy.
Mental health	Like the community services arrangement, there is usually a fixed element based on historic costs and activity. A variable element can be linked to identified mental health resource groups, and likewise a further quality element could be applied for agreed activities with a quality focus. Risk share elements could be designed to address high-cost patients who require intensive support and/or residential stays. A locally agreed price can apply, with upper and lower thresholds to manage the risks for commissioner and provider.
Voluntary, community and social enterprise	A good example of a VCSE local blended payment arrangement is hospice care. A blended payment approach can be used to strengthen and support the often-complex arrangements with hospice providers. Hospices often provide a mix of traditionally NHS-funded care and non-NHS social and holistic support. In this scenario, the NHS commissioner may agree a fixed payment in support of some or all the activity that is typically NHS-funded care. The variable element may consist of a quality-based arrangement that incentivises good outcomes for people. These outcomes may be a result of a mixture of traditional and non-traditional care and support, which is usually personalised and holistic in nature. In these arrangements, the hospices receive a share of funding that contributes to their sustainability.

Social care funding arrangements

Social care funding is very different from NHS arrangements. Social care is a devolved policy area, which means that decisions are not led by a national body but are instead made at a local level by local government. Social care is the biggest spend area for local authorities.

A key difference is the mechanism of financial contribution made by some people receiving social care. The NHS is free at the point of use, but publicly funded social care is not freely available to all. Some people make a contribution to costs where they have financial assets. These contributions are in the main applicable for homecare and residential care.

These differences are a potential issue for individuals when the lines between social care and health care blur. Many people require a mixture of both types of care when they have complex health, social care, and mental health needs. Holistic care encompasses physical, emotional, social, and spiritual needs, so joint working for the NHS and social care is vital to achieving those aims. The integrated care systems will go some way to supporting joint working, but consideration of how funding approaches will align is required. Joint commissioning and continuing healthcare are two examples of bridging the gap in funding approaches.

Joint commissioning

The Health Act 2006 introduced Section 75, a mechanism whereby a local authority and health commissioning organisation can implement a partnership of equal control. Section 75 provides for delegation of a local authority's health-related functions to its NHS partner, and vice versa, to meet shared objectives and create joint funding arrangements. This is referred to as **joint commissioning**.

Joint commissioning benefits include:

- supporting discharge pathways and avoiding delays;
- reducing pressure on acute and emergency services;
- improving capacity and capability of intermediate care;
- accelerating integration and improvement programmes;
- strengthening a collaborative culture;
- developing workforce capacity, skills, and joint working arrangements;
- implementing system-wide recovery plans and initiatives.

In real terms, this can result in collaboration for wide population benefits, such as targeted commissioning for a specific need or a common challenge, like improving outcomes for people with learning disabilities or people who are homeless. Organisations can pool or align budgets so that funding is maximised and its use is transparent. In addition to funding, joint commissioning approaches can share workforce, skills, and expertise to improve outcomes. Joint commissioning tends to be values based, and it aims to co-produce with people, reduce inequalities, and increase social value.

On a less positive note, all the many benefits aside, it is important to be aware that joint commissioning often takes a lot of time, as working with multiple partners, agendas, governance structures, and so on will slow the process down, and the benefits may take time to realise. In fact, in some cases, the approach may cost more, as unmet need is identified. Realistic aims and objectives will be helpful to the approach and robust evaluation will in many cases evidence it was worth the effort.

Where NHS healthcare services are commissioned under these joint commissioning arrangements, they remain in the scope of the 2023/25 NHS Payment Scheme, even if predominantly commissioned by a local authority. Therefore, the same payment rules would apply to the provider in question.

Continuing healthcare

Continuing healthcare is discussed here, as it is a provision of great cost with responsibilities shared between health and social care commissioners. NHS continuing healthcare is free healthcare provided by the NHS to individuals with ongoing healthcare needs. A package of care is funded for any setting – for example, the person's own home, a care home, or a hospice. Patient needs are the key factor, not location. The healthcare need must be primarily health related (not a social care need), ongoing (not temporary), and substantial, and it is often complex. Where these conditions are met, then full costs are covered by the NHS, with the patient having no obligation to contribute.

For people under the age of 18, the process is very similar, and it is referred to as 'NHS Continuing Care'.

'Fast track' refers to the rapid implementation of continuing healthcare or continuing care where it is likely a person is nearing the end of their life. This ensures rapid care is offered without delays of lengthy assessments and bureaucracy.

Although continuing healthcare and continuing care funding is for a health need, the people receiving it very often need support and care for social needs too. This is due to the complexity and severity of their need. Therefore, when a continuing healthcare or continuing care panel meet to discuss cases and agree eligibility, a social care representative is a key and equal member. This representative agree the social needs identified for each case, and then in partnership the parties agree the split of costs between NHS and local authority. A multidisciplinary team, comprised of health and social care professionals, will have already completed an assessment of the patient, and this informs the panel.

Alternative funding models

Although most of acute care is bound by the NHS Payment Scheme terms, the mental health and community provider contracts usually have flexibility to examine other approaches that can be applied within the NHS Payment Scheme framework – for example, as a variable, quality-based, or risk-sharing element. These examples include outcomes-based approaches, community and mental health currency frameworks, and personal health budgets, though others exist too.

Outcomes-based funding

Outcomes-based financial arrangements are essentially a method of seeking quality and cost-effectiveness. The more effective a service is at achieving its aim, the more funding it will attract. The greater the benefit, the stronger the justification for the expenditure. (I discuss the advantages and pitfalls of identifying and evaluating outcomes more fully in Chapter 8.)

In the blended payment approach, to incentivise quality commissioners can apply a quality-based variable element. The proportion of this variable element in comparison to the overall contract value will vary depending on factors such as how much of the contract activity is aligned with that particular objective, how large the contract value is, or how much risk there is to the provider if they don't achieve the objective. Therefore, commissioners could apply a low or high percentage to the agreed quality-based element.

Examples of what a quality-based variable outcome could include are reduced patient blood pressure levels, completion of a personalised care and support plan, improved patient-reported pain levels, and satisfaction of support among families whose loved ones are at the end of life. The outcomes don't have to be directly linked to patients and their families though. Other areas to consider might include application of shared packages of care across providers, training and development of staff, or referrals to other services, such as social prescribing. These would all realise indirect quality outcomes.

These approaches have similarities with CQUIN targets. Therefore, learning from CQUIN targets can be applied. For example, don't overvalue this proportion. If there is too much financial risk wrapped up in the arrangement, then other areas of the service may suffer as frustrated providers focus all their energies on one area. Similarly, keep the outcome aim ambitious but achievable. If the aim is not far-reaching enough, there is no real benefit gained; likewise, if it is too ambitious, the provider may give up before they have begun. Finally, make the outcome aim meaningful and linked to wider strategic priorities – this adds to the impetus for achievement if providers see how they are contributing to a wide system-based improvement in quality.

Community currencies

NHS England has been working closely with partners since 2017 to develop currencies for specific populations (NHS England, 2021b). The development of needs-based currencies for community services offers an opportunity to move towards evidence-based pricing, which supports a person-centred approach and proactive care management. A currency is not a price – it is a unit to which a local price can be applied. Where everyone uses the same currency units, it is easier to compare and contrast costs and performance. The prices that are applied to the units can reflect local costs and arrangements.

In 2021, NHS England shared currency models for 'frailty' and 'last year of life' (LYOL). These currencies have been developed to support implementation of several different payment options, ranging from payment aligned to patient pathways or patient-based budgets. The publication of these currencies for non-mandatory use in 2021/22 was the first step in a larger programme to develop currencies and payment mechanisms for community-based services which support a whole-system approach. The implementation of community currencies will support benchmarking between providers, aid collaboration, and assist the commissioning process.

An example of the currency model, for LYOL, is provided in Table 7.4 – this is taken from the NHS England community services currency guidance. Eleven LYOL currencies are shown. These currencies are made up of a person's phase of illness, from stable to deceased, and this is combined with a person's functional status. Here, the Australian modified Karnofsky performance scale is used. This defines a person's status according to three categories – high, medium, and low – broken down in Table 7.5.

By combining the illness phase and functional status of a person, providers and commissioners can better identify and predict what

Table 7.4: Last year of life currencies

Currency unit	Phase of illness	Functional status*
LYOL_1	Stable	Low
LYOL_2	Stable	Medium
LYOL_3	Stable	High
LYOL_4	Unstable	Low
LYOL_5	Unstable	Medium
LYOL_6	Unstable	High
LYOL_7	Deteriorating	Low
LYOL_8	Deteriorating	Medium
LYOL_9	Deteriorating	High
LYOL_10	Dying	
LYOL_11	Deceased	

Note: * based on the Australian modified Karnofsky scale

Source: NHS England (2021b)

Table 7.5: Australian modified Karnofsky scale

	Score	Descriptor
High	100%	Normal; no complaints; no evidence of disease
	90%	Able to carry on normal activity; minor signs or symptoms of disease
	80%	Normal activity with effort; some signs or symptoms of disease
Medium	70%	Cares for self; unable to carry on normal activities or to do active work
	60%	Requires assistance but is able to care for most personal needs
	50%	Requires considerable assistance and frequent medical care
Low	40%	In bed more than 50% of the time
	30%	Almost completely bedfast
	20%	Totally bedfast and requiring extensive nursing care by professionals and/or family
	10%	Comatose or barely rousable
	0%	Dead

Source: NHS England (2021b)

their needs may be, plus what they may need next, which is useful for forward planning. Patients are regularly reviewed, and their status updated accordingly. A local unit price can be agreed for each currency, to more accurately reflect the actual costs of meeting the person's health and wellbeing needs.

Using currencies in this way can improve the quality of data collection and subsequently the process of agreeing accurate and fair fixed elements of contracts. It also allows for comparison with similar providers – for example, across community service providers or hospices – and therefore supports benchmarking.

Both the LYOL and the frailty currencies are under continued development as of 2023/24. The currency teams are also working with partners to develop similar models for children and young people with disabilities, long-term conditions, and single episodes of care.

Mental health resource groups

Like the community currencies, mental health resource groups aim to group patients according to classifications. The improved understanding of mental health activity and patient need will, like the community currencies, support identification of needs and how they are addressed. It will also contribute to attaining parity of funding and development with physical healthcare.

Clustering groups of people with care needs has been in place since 2012, but it was recognised in 2021 that there was a need to improve the system and develop a more meaningful set of groups for mental health services to use. The intention was to use the Patient Level Information Costing System (PLICS) and SNOMED CT terminology (see Chapter 4) to improve the quality and granularity of data collected. An example of new groups is shown in Figure 7.3. In this example, the patient's disorder type, the severity level, and the intervention are combined to create a mental health resource group. The grouping would be regularly reviewed by a clinician to ensure it is still appropriate. The cross-cutting sections are driven by type of service rather than by disorder, and they include crisis and secure care services.

This model was under development at the time of writing and consultation will shape the format and delivery of this framework for quality data collection and associated funding models.

Good to know: Patient Level Information and Costing System

PLICS data information tools collect and analyse patient-level data, especially information about cost. PLICS data is collected and used by acute, mental health, ambulance, community, and talking therapies providers.

The data is used for improvements, but the main aim is to examine and compare costs of provision. It can assist providers to maximise resources, identify efficiencies, and carry out benchmarking. It can help identify unwarranted variation, match the actual costs of services to any national tariffs or currencies, and increased understanding of effective and efficient care models.

The providers use **information standards** to ensure that everybody is collecting the same data in the same way. This makes comparisons meaningful.

Figure 7.3: Mental health resource groups

Disorder group	A. Psychotic disorders & bipolars*	B. Common mental health disorders	C. Personality disorders	D. Eating disorders	E. Organic mental disorders
Severity level	(A1) **Mild**	(B1) **Mild**	(C1) **Mild**	(D1) **Mild**	(E1) **Mild**
	(A2) **Moderate**	(B2) **Moderate**	(C2) **Moderate**	(D2) **Moderate**	(E2) **Moderate**
	(A3) **Severe**	(B3) **Severe**	(C3) **Severe**	(D3) **Severe**	(E3) **Severe**
Cross cutting settings (common across disorder groups)	(F) Crisis care	Crisis care	Crisis care *Crisis care*	Crisis care	Crisis care
	(G) Secure care	Secure care	Secure care *Secure care*	Secure care	Secure care

*Includes affective and non-affective disorders, can be split into two groups if clinically appropriate
*Will also consider relevance of MHRGs for perinatal mental health services and CYP MH

17 MHRGs

Source: NHS England and NHS Improvement (2020) Open Government Licence v3.0

PLICS is a useful tool to use when examining the cost of a current pathway and comparing it to a cost of a new pathway or service. In this way, commissioners and providers can provide evidence that a different approach may be more cost-effective. For example, PLICS can show how much it costs for patients to have multiple consultations and investigations across several specialties rather than a one-stop model with a multidisciplinary team.

Personal health budgets

I consider the benefits and when to use personal health budgets in Chapter 10. Here, I outline the financial side of these mechanisms of payment.

A personal health budget is an amount of money identified to support the health and wellbeing needs of a particular patient. The budget, and what it aims to improve or manage, is planned and agreed between that patient and their professional. The aim is to empower the patient to use the money that would have been spent on them with traditional care but in a different way that better suits their individual needs.

Deciding the amount of money allocated to each person in a personal health budget is a separate and individual exercise. An initial budget is set, followed by a conversation between the person and a professional to develop a personalised care and support plan (see more in Chapter 10). The initial budget value is guided by what is needed to support the person and any local commissioning parameters. The personal health budget value should be set at no more than the cost of care that the person would have received under traditionally commissioned services. Personal health budgets should not cost commissioners more, though occasionally needs may be identified that were missed in traditional pathways. There is an argument that supporting these people to use personal health budgets not only improves their health and wellbeing, but saves on future health costs that may have occurred if they were not supported adequately.

The initial budget-setting process is important, because there is a need to (NHS England, 2019b):

- support people to adequately plan and make decisions about their care – people need to know the amount of money in their budget;

- have a consistent approach to budget setting to ensure fairness across all budget holders;
- understand costs at a person level and plan for the population accordingly.

Done well, the initial budget-setting conversation will be transparent so that the person and those close to them are aware of what the budget is for, how it has been calculated, and how much it is. This should be done before the support is planned in detail.

Commissioners usually offer personal health budgets where there are legal rights to do so and for a distinct set of other locally agreed needs (Chapter 10 has more details). There is often a simple framework in place to help assign an indicative budget that matches a person's needs. The budgets are informed by historical costs. If more complex arrangements are required, perhaps with multiple services or organisations, all the cost information can be brought together in one place, enabling the development of one budget with different elements. In this way, joint working may be identified. Likewise, health and social care budgets can be pooled in an **integrated budget** to align care and support more effectively. A **statement of resources** is a tool that brings all the activity and cost information together for health, social care, and education. It summarises this information to ease the processes of budget setting across organisations. The usual process is for an integrated care board-delegated group to sign off the final personal health budget.

There are three types of personal health budget:

- With a **notional budget**, no money changes hands, and the patient and a nominated professional agree how to spend the money. Then the NHS arranges the agreed care. This arrangement is an easy option for the patient, as they do not need to manage the administrative burden. It is still a personal budget approach, as the patient has chosen this approach above others. An example might be a person choosing a particular wheelchair provider. (Note: If an integrated care board uses a notional budget to pay providers of NHS services, this is in the scope of the NHS Payment Scheme. Therefore, the payment will be governed by the rules applicable to the services in question.)

- A **real budget** can be held by a third party, which is an organisation legally independent of the patient and their NHS commissioner. This third party will hold the budget and pay for the care in the agreed care plan.
- A **direct payment** is where the budget is transferred to the patient (or their nominated carer) to buy the care that has been agreed between the person and their NHS commissioner. The patient or carer will then enact the contracts or payments for the necessary services.

The integrated care board will ensure that all three types of personal health budget are offered where appropriate in the circumstances. Where there is choice in terms of the type of budget, a person would be supported with the right information to make an informed choice. For example, continuing healthcare arrangements could be arranged via a real budget with the independent body organising and paying for care; or the patient might choose a direct payment approach with the patient or carer making the arrangements and making payments themselves. It should also be possible for people to change the method as they go through the process if they wish.

As would be expected, there are some rules about who and how money can be offered directly to patients. For example, it may be unsuitable for some people to receive a direct payment and alternatives such as real budgets will be more appropriate. And there is often concern that people will spend the money on things that were not part of their plan. However, this seems to be a very rare occurrence and it should not concern commissioners enough to remove the benefits of personal health budgets. If it does occur, then commissioners can remove the right to a direct payment and offer an alternative.

Individual funding requests

Individual funding requests are cases where a patient and their clinician ask the integrated care board to pay for a specific treatment that is not routinely funded. A treatment is not routinely funded for several reasons, but more commonly the treatment is either not proven to be very effective, too expensive compared to other treatments, or experimental. Despite these reasons, a clinician may feel that a patient has certain clinical exceptionality that means they would benefit from the treatment.

To make an individual funding request application, there must be evidence of clinical exceptionality – that is, what makes that patient clinically different from others. This exceptionality would potentially mean the patient would benefit more than others. No non-clinical factors, such as family commitments or ability to work, are taken into account.

A panel sits to discuss each case. If agreed as appropriate to fund, there would be no formal contracting arrangement already in place to pay for this treatment, as it is not routinely funded. Therefore, a cost per case arrangement would apply with an agreed one-off price applied. As this money must be found from somewhere, the funding usually comes from the budget that the alternative treatment would have come from. If the cost of the treatment is paid to a low-volume activity contract provider, both parties need to be aware that subsequent year averages may be higher due to this one-off activity cost or that it can be pushed above the £500,000 threshold, in which case the next year a contract is required. No invoicing can take place outside of the low-volume activity arrangement.

Good to know: National Institute for Health and Care Excellence

As medical technology advances, many new treatments, medicines, equipment, and surgical techniques become available every year. Some of these are introduced into the NHS in response to guidance from the National Institute for Health and Care Excellence (NICE).

NICE helps commissioners purchase the best care while ensuring safety and value for money. They do this by:

• assessing the evidence of new technologies and medicines for safety, efficacy, and value for money;
• producing resources for guidance, policies, and quality standards;
• proving recommendations on innovation for priorities and promoting best practice.

When examining any health or social care area for improvement, it is important to refer to the latest NICE guidance. It is well respected by commissioners, providers, and the public and should be implemented wherever possible, but it is not mandatory. (See the NICE website for more: www.nice.org.uk/)

Finding the money

One of the biggest challenges for commissioners is the struggle to find the money for new investment or improvements to services. The health and wellbeing need is often clearly demonstrated, but with so many competing priorities and increasingly limited funds, how do you find the money to meet all the priorities? It is a problem to which there is no simple answer, but there are usually options. I have provided a few pointers, which can be considered when trying to 'find the money'.

Invest to save

All funding for services that is new or increased needs to be justified. If, in addition to benefits for patients, commissioners can also demonstrate that a change is likely to save money, then they have a stronger case for change. 'Invest to save' (spending money to accrue more money) is a term commonly used. The idea is that by spending money in one area you can release even more money elsewhere is not new. The premise is that money is recouped, and the cost of the service is outweighed by the savings made.

For example, a self-management programme for diabetes would seek to empower patients to effectively measure and manage their own insulin levels. Their insulin would be better controlled, and they would be less likely to be admitted to Accident and Emergency, develop retinopathy, or require surgery for limb amputations – all of which are costly care episodes or interventions. The cost of a self-management programme with support from a community diabetes service will be far lower than the cost of the complications that can arise. This is a strong example, but there are many to be found with preventative care as their focus.

Another approach to invest to save is redesigning services to remove repetition or unnecessary steps. An example here may be a one-stop service with a multidisciplinary team for complex and unexplained symptoms – this team would be expensive to implement but would be overall cheaper than several pathways cross-referring the same patient to each other to perform multiple investigations and treatments that may have been avoidable with a single team approach.

Prevention

Prevention streams can be delivered within the wider community. It may be difficult to justify funding for these when there are so many immediate health and social care priorities to address, but even small investments in prevention can have a big impact. Estimates vary but it is generally accepted that 10–20 per cent of the wider determinants of health are shaped by healthcare (Fytche, 2023); therefore, 80–90 per cent sit with the wider system. This is an enormous amount of potential impact, so there is value in shaping prevention interventions within the integrated care system. This could be a system-wide approach of looking at population health and future planning. For example, implementing sustainable funding to the voluntary, community and social enterprise (VCSE) sector to apply a joined-up approach to prevention and self-care activities would in years to come reap benefits of reduced incidence of disease or illness. A gradual shift in resources, to match the maturity of VCSE capacity and confidence, will likely improve outcomes and reduce demand on NHS and social care services.

Repurposing

This is a method of using the funds already available with no new investment – it's not popular with providers for obvious reasons, but it can be an effective solution when used in a targeted way.

Disinvesting for change

This repurposing option involves replacing one service with another, so the money is being used in a new way. An example is ending a single consultant-led clinic and replacing it with a supervised multiple-nurse practitioner clinic – in this scenario, it is important to be mindful of the risks and implications of 'stopping' a service. The new service must be considered cost-effective and safe, and it must deliver on quality outcomes to be worth the upheaval of change.

Using vacancy factors

This is an often-overlooked option, but where providers are transparent, they can share details of currently unused funds, which are often due to staff vacancies. This is a less complex way of repurposing funds, and it allows incremental changes with less upheaval for staff and services. An example is using the funds from staff vacancies to implement a self-management approach which requires less staff input. Improved self-management skills among patients would reduce the need for follow-ups, which in turn leads to less staff time being taken up. As the self-management outcomes become apparent, there can be further step changes in the development of the service.

Top slicing budgets

In this scenario, the commissioner encourages an approach of collaboration. Taking a small proportion of an identified provider budget and specifying how this is to be used in a different way can be catalyst for change.

There have been a few instances with health contracts where the contract budget is top-sliced by a small percentage, say 2–4 per cent, and there is an expectation of investment of those funds with the VCSE sector. This funded VCSE provision would support the work already provided by the main provider, and the partnerships and pathways between the organisations would be strengthened with the benefits of improved outcomes. For example, a children's mental health provider has 2 per cent top-sliced from their budget, which the provider must invest in VCSE organisations that can provide services for the children and young people. This could be support while waiting for an assessment, peer groups, or parent support groups.

Social investment

Social investment is the use of repayable finance to help an organisation achieve a social purpose. It is often used to develop new or existing activities for a variety of outcomes, such as prevention of illness and improvement of health and wellbeing. The money can come from different sources, including impact investors, such as Macmillan Cancer Support and Big Society Capital. These impact investors provide upfront funding with no guarantee of return. A fund manager, such as Social Finance, would work with the receiving body to design and implement lasting change using the funds. Repayment is made as outcomes are realised, and the preventative approach will support long-term benefits for public services.

Social impact bonds and social outcomes contracts are mechanisms that apply social investment. They are like an outcomes-based contract developed to tackle a social or environmental challenge. The flexibility they offer provides freedom to test new approaches with less financial risk.

Social Finance is one group that have been championing the approach, and they have supported multiple projects to fruition. Several examples of successful application of the approach, including significant work within palliative and end of life care, can be found on their website (see www.socialfinance.org.uk/what-we-do/projects).

As they and others have proven the potential for social investment on an individual service level, there are prospects for the approach to support integrated care system-wide innovation funding, with enabled transformation and improved patient care.

Katy Nex (2023) from Social Finance points out that 'the Hewitt review called for 1 per cent of the NHS budget to focus on prevention, while acknowledging there is no new money to support this shift. NHS leadership knows this is the right thing to do, but there is little opportunity to invest, test, and learn.' Social investment can provide these opportunities, and every integrated care system should be aiming to have a range of social investment projects within their local plans for development.

Efficiencies

Unfortunately, we will not anytime soon be able to escape the never-ending need for more and more efficiencies of working. The public sector is likely to continue to suffer with limited resources and the NHS and social care will continue to have new initiatives placed on them to save more money. For example, at the time of writing, Prime Minister Rishi Sunak has announced a 15-year NHS Long Term Workforce Plan (NHS England, 2023e) to reform the NHS, with the promise of additional training places and more. However, the trade-off is an ask of further efficiencies, with a range of 1.5–2 per cent higher levels of productivity through a range of opportunities. Putting aside exasperation at the call for more cost-cutting, there are opportunities in the efficiencies suggested in this plan; plus there are others to consider, such as:

- provider collaboratives – savings on back office functions and shared key workforce across teams;
- care closer to home – investing in primary, community, physical, and mental health services and the VCSE sector will reduce more expensive care in the acute sector. Other initiatives can include moving hospital admissions to hospital at home or moving treatments from theatres to outpatient settings;
- increased training of generalist staff – to reduce burden on specialist clinicians;
- medical and operational advancement for productivity – examples include moving to more day case procedures rather than overnight stays, or less invasive surgical techniques;
- efficiencies at scale – partnerships between organisations across a wider locality or regional footprint where services have low volume and/or high costs.

These and other ideas for efficiencies will be identified and implemented more effectively when done in partnership. Commissioners can ensure that professionals, who are often best placed for designing innovation, have limited barriers to suggesting and implementing efficiency improvements.

Match funding and pump-priming

This approach is frequently used by NHS England and regional commissioners to help new developments get off the ground. **Match funding** is where a total value of funding is split proportionally between two bodies. For example, 50 per cent of the total cost would be shared by each party. This approach can be useful in many ways – for example **pump-priming**. Pump-priming is an approach where a new initiative has an injection of funding to get it started – often for long enough to prove it works well. Then when the evidence of success is captured, the substantive funding can be justified for longer-term delivery. For example, the NHS England children and young people's palliative and end of life care match funding scheme from 2019 to 2024 offered 50 per cent of total funding to eligible commissioners, who then used this financial top-up to gain traction on much-needed developments. The idea was to create sustainability in the sector, as commissioners could pump-prime change and evidence the benefits for longer-term local investment.

This was a national scheme, but the approach can be used locally. Match funding can be used by integrated care boards that wish to support VCSE initiatives in receipt of charitable funding. This could be used so that VCSE providers kick-start or improve local community assets and provision. There is a sharing of financial risk between the parties. West Suffolk Council did this when they launched a match funding scheme for community action on climate change (West Suffolk Council, 2022). They offered £150,000 in total for VCSE organisations to bid on. The successful project bids would receive 50 per cent of their costs up to £10,000. This collective action empowered communities, increased motivation, and led a movement in tackling the climate emergency in their locality.

Pump-priming funds can be offered to almost any provider with innovative ideas. The temporary funds will support the costs of change. Recurrent funding can then be identified as either an older alternative activity is phased out or the realised savings are reinvested. For example, a provider wants to develop a one-stop clinic with a multidisciplinary team for complex medical symptoms in children. There is a start-up cost with training and administration to develop the new approach. There is no additional money available, but the model promises to save costs on consultations, investigations, procedures, and admissions. The commissioner offers a one-off sum to implement the initiative for two years. The evaluation shows evidence of savings, and this service becomes recurrent at no extra cost to the commissioner in the long term.

Micro-commissioning grants

Micro-commissioning involves small and proportionate amounts for improving local service offers. These are primarily small grants awarded to VCSE providers to support and enable community-based assets and services.

At its heart is a reduced administrative and governance approach to remove barriers for those offering services or assets in the community, plus small and manageable financial commitments for the commissioner.

The grants are quick and easy to implement, and the sums of money are small. Although these approaches may not address large-scale priorities, they can strengthen and expand the formally commissioned health and social care services.

An example of use can be seen with social prescribing. I examine social prescribing aims and implementation more closely in Chapter 10, but the approach often involves many small community initiatives, such as hobby groups, informal support groups, and so on. There must be some micro-governance to ensure safety for people who are 'referred', but this cannot be a barrier or challenge for those offering activities. Very simple grants and communication arrangements, perhaps through a VCSE conduit, can provide assurance for commissioners while supporting a thriving community.

REFLECTIONS FOR LEADERS

Balancing the books with the Elective Recovery Fund

In 2023/24, £2.5 billion is earmarked for the Elective Recovery Fund, with the intention of restoring balance after the world-wide pandemic. This has been allocated to integrated care boards on a fair share basis. But during 2023/24, and in subsequent years, the boards will be struggling to deliver what the Elective Recovery Fund intends, as the system grapples with staffing shortages, strikes, and very tight budgets.

This sweeping focus on elective activity for the blended payment model is very restrictive and it does not fit the aims of the NHS Payment Scheme to ease and simplify payment of providers. Payment for all elective activity at a unit price feels very much like the (former) National Tariff. It could be a costly approach for commissioners as integrated care boards must pay for all elective activity delivered. The plan does not take into consideration the activity that must take place outside of hospital, such as the primary care or community services that may be affected by this push on clearing the backlog of cases. Where is the whole-system support? And mental health waits have also suffered during the pandemic – how can these be prioritised too?

Talking to neighbouring integrated care boards and regional and national colleagues about how to tackle these issues will help those with the unenviable act of balancing the books in the next few years.

Suggestions for success

A common issue facing commissioning today is the lack of available funding. While the national payment system will aim to ease some large-scale funding issues, it gets trickier to balance the books when considering competing local needs. Transparency is key – share the difficult decisions you make with your partners and invite innovative thinking to finance and enable change. Be wary of paying for 'cheap' services – buying something for less is not always good value.

Negotiating finance is always a potential threat to relationships between commissioner and provider. Relationships can be left in tatters. You may find it helpful to pre-agree some overarching principles before starting. These could include a shared vision for improving outcomes, maintaining a respectful relationship, transparency, and so on. These could be part of the contracting intentions document. The sharing of the intention to remain on good and effective terms is an enabler for agreeing a financial plan without the tension.

8

Evaluating impact

Aim

This chapter looks at how to design evaluation that is effective at measuring impact and outcomes, and can inform the commissioning cycle process. The types of evaluation and how to feed evaluation findings into the commissioning cycle are discussed. As not all evaluations show good outcomes, what to do with poor performance or outcomes is considered.

What are we measuring?

To ensure they have achieved what they set out to do, commissioners must evaluate the **outcomes** and **outputs** of a service. Outcomes are the benefits realised by an action or series of actions. Measuring outcomes ensures real results are being achieved for people and that what is being done is working. Outputs are the activities and steps taken. Measuring outputs allows commissioners and providers to demonstrate that the activities put into place can be attributed to the successful outcomes. Outcomes are the 'what' you want to achieve, and the outputs are the 'how'.

We measure and evaluate the success of services in order to:

- ensure delivery of plans;
- confirm if the service is a success or failure:
  - o if a success, evaluation can inform spread and scale;

      o if a failure, there is a need to correct or replace;
      o for either success or failure, there is value in sharing the learning;
- demonstrate results and win stakeholder support and confidence;
- be accountable to regulators;
- demonstrate value with taxpayer money.

Good evaluation will examine not just operationality and ability for churning out activity, but a range of factors that indicate true success. Effective evaluation measures consider whether the activity is:

- delivering any benefits;
- value for money;
- safe;
- accessible to all who need it;
- delivering a good experience for people;
- supporting and enabling a confident workforce;
- sustainable;
- creating unintended consequences;
- meeting national standards;
- offering benefits with societal value.

Outcome measures are now rightly considered the epitome of evaluation for health and wellbeing initiatives. When we refer to outcomes, we are including a range of factors. As seen in the earlier list, success is wider than an outcome for an individual, important as that may be. Outcomes need to encompass benefits for a population, for the community, and for the system, to enable it to continue operating effectively. Therefore, outcome measures are defined here as consequences for a range of beneficiaries, in a range of ways, but one of the most important beneficiaries remains the patient – this is, of course, fundamental in healthcare.

And although outcome measures are commonly used, you cannot fully assess success without considering process and structural indicators too. These can seem more bureaucratic, but they are important elements, especially for large-scale services or those with more risk associated with them. This combined approach gives a fuller assessment of benefits, progress, sustainability, and safety. It also helps guide where improvements can be made and where to target action.

The key elements for evaluation are described next. Every service or change being evaluated will need a targeted approach to designing the right metrics – these can be chosen from those shared in Table 8.1.

Table 8.1: Types of evaluation measure

Indicator type	Benefits	Collection and analysis
Structural	These indicators include elements such as infrastructure or provider-level systems that have an impact on the quality of care. Examples include: • staffing levels; • staffing qualifications and training; • surgical volumes; • access to equipment. These can be more predictive of performance than outcomes, but they have an impact on both.	The data are usually readily available and inexpensive to collect.
Process	These indicators relate to pathways or processes, such as: • an offer of preventative services, like cancer screening; • time-related processes, like a scan within 24 hours of a stroke; • waiting times for treatment; • discharge processes, like prescribing statins after cardiac admissions. These are often good indicators of quality for specific conditions and disease management.	These are often evidence-based indicators and a direct measure of quality. They are easily measured and interpreted, but can be too specific and narrow. A common complaint is that data collection becomes a 'tick box' exercise with no real meaningful analysis of actual outcomes for people.
Clinical outcomes	These indicators reflect the patient's result. They can be final outcomes, such as amputation, or intermediate outcomes, such as insulin control. There are numerous other examples, including: • hospital admission rates; • deaths from cancer; • blood pressure control; • healthy births.	These reflect all the factors influencing a patient's care. They are easy to measure and can be easy to attribute to good care in the acute sector, but more difficult to link to care received in primary and community settings. There can be a time lag between the care and the outcome, and the outcomes can be affected by factors outside of direct care.

(continued)

Table 8.1: Types of evaluation measure (continued)

Indicator type	Benefits	Collection and analysis
	These are more practically applied with some health conditions than others. Not all health conditions will have such a clearly defined outcome.	
Patient-reported outcome measures	These are outcomes reported by the patient. There are nationally set patient-reported outcome measures, such as for hip replacements or varicose vein surgery – or you can develop local measures to allow patients to report their own outcomes. For example, a patient questionnaire exploring their health and wellbeing after completing a rehabilitation course. These measures commonly include symptoms, pain, mobility, and wellbeing.	Nationally set patient-reported outcome measures have guidance for collection and are easily comparable. Locally designed measures will vary but it is a good idea to ensure that the parameters given to the patient for reporting are specific and not onerous to complete.
Achievement of patient goals	Like patient-reported outcome measures, these indicators are reliant on patient reporting. These specifically measure if a patient-set goal has been achieved. The goals will differ between various diseases, procedures, health and wellbeing status before illness or procedure, and the patient's preferences. For example, one person would like to return to running marathons after knee surgery, while another patient may wish to return to walking their grandchild to school without pain.	Often these goals are confirmed as part of the personalised care and support planning conversation (see Chapter 10). After a pre-agreed period, the patient is asked to report if they have achieved their personal goal in full, in part, or not at all. This can be subjective, but it is an easy measure to collect and record. Care must be taken that goals are realistic but appropriately ambitious.
Patient-reported experience measures	These are experiences reported by the patient. Like patient-reported outcome measures, they require a patient to complete an assessment of their own experience. This can include elements such as compassion (respect, dignity, and empathy), communication (information provided, choice, consent, and shared decision	These can and should be part of routine assessment. Questionnaires should be readily available and easy to understand and complete. Today electronic questionnaires are commonly used.

Table 8.1: Types of evaluation measure (continued)

Indicator type	Benefits	Collection and analysis
	making), timeliness (waiting times, cancellations, responsiveness to queries), and reliability (safety, dependability, acting on results or symptoms).	
Cost-effectiveness	This is the analysis of the cost of delivering a service balanced against the changes in health outcomes. The difficult part is deciding what cost value is worth a particular rise in health improvements. If a service is very expensive but creates significant improvements in health, then it can be deemed cost-effective; a service that is very cheap to run but has no discernible health benefits will have low cost-effectiveness.	A simple way of analysing cost-effectiveness is to consider what costs are avoided or reduced by implementing the change. These are often proxy measures, as it is difficult to count the cost of what hasn't happened, but a baseline of costs collected before the change was implemented can be a helpful comparator to assess cost impacts. Services with holistic approaches are more difficult to assess financially – it is usually appropriate to estimate the preventative benefits and the health and wellbeing outcomes and balance these against the costs of implementation.
Cost-effectiveness of voluntary, community and social enterprise services	Social return on investment is a common mechanism of attributing value to VCSE activity or services. This is usually expressed as a return on investment per pound spent. For example, a case study presented by the Department of Health (2010) shows that a housing and rehabilitation service for families following drug abuse had a potential return of £2.83 for every £1 invested.	This approach uses proxy measures of estimated avoided costs to demonstrate the financial value of investment in the community. Savings are often across a range of organisations.
Social value	Social value indicators are a range of factors to demonstrate benefit across a whole system. They include social, economic, and environmental indicators, and	These are often high-level approximations of what benefits could be realised.

(continued)

Table 8.1: Types of evaluation measure (continued)

Indicator type	Benefits	Collection and analysis
	general wellbeing of an area. They might also be indicators for creation of new jobs, economic growth, outcome of activities to tackle climate change, or outcome of activities to develop communities.	
Equity	These are not direct indicators of quality or outcomes, but they have an indirect effect. Monitoring should include assessment of different population groups and include: • variations in access; • variations in quality; • severity of disease at point of contact; • clinical outcomes; • patient experience.	Collection of demographic data aids the analysis, but this needs to be supported by collection of patient voices for assessment of patient experience.

Evaluation metrics: An illustration

An example of how these measures can be applied to a particular service is shared here. Any number of measures can be used in evaluation, and those used in the example are by no means exhaustive, but ten is about the right number of measures for a new service – that gives a balance of evaluating effectively without it becoming a burden.

The example is an evaluation of a diabetes service with integration of both community and voluntary, community and social enterprise (VCSE) providers.

The measures used for evaluation are:

- structural – percentage of generalist workforce (nurses and allied health professionals) who receive training in diabetes management;
- process – percentage of people offered the self-management programme within 14 days of diagnosis;
- process – percentage of people who agree a personalised care and support plan;

- clinical outcomes – percentage of people with a safe level of insulin at annual review;
- patient-reported outcome measures – percentage of people reporting they feel more confident managing their own condition;
- patient goals – percentage of people who have achieved weight loss goals;
- patient-reported experience measures – percentage of people reporting they have timely contact from professionals;
- cost-effectiveness:
  o number of emergency admissions for diabetes compared to baseline data;
  o return on investment of VCSE services: cost-effectiveness compared against admissions, Accident and Emergency attendances, consultant first and follow-up attendances;
- equity – a demographic breakdown of the data to compare socioeconomic groups accessing the services.

Good to know: Friends and family test

The friends and family test is a national initiative that is used as a feedback tool for patient experience. It supports the process of listening to patients and helps identify what is working well and what needs improvement.

The test asks patients about their experience in a manner that is quick and simple. It is designed to be an anonymous process, and it is completed at a time convenient for the patient. There is at least one default question accompanied by a limited number of responses, and then there is opportunity for patients to share their thoughts in their own words in a space for free text. Providers can use the free text space to frame any particular question that is helpful to them.

As well as providers and local commissioners, NHS England use the test for quality improvement work and the Care Quality Commission use it during their inspections.

As it offers a continuous source of data, partners can use this to examine trends over time – for example, to see if there is improvement in experience after a new service or pathway is launched. The data is a very high-level indicator of patient satisfaction, and to get a true understanding of patient experience, more specific tools need to be employed. (See more on the test at: www.england.nhs.uk/fft/.)

Key performance indicators

Key performance indicators (KPIs) are evaluation measures frequently used with high-value contracts. KPIs tend to be specifically connected to performance and have less of a focus on outcomes. They are often linked to process measures (see Table 8.1). Examples of KPIs are the percentage of patients who have their first appointment within ten days of referral and the percentage of patients who are discharged within five days. There are advantages in including KPIs alongside outcome measures where the KPI in question has a close correlation with process and experience.

KPIs come with **targets** and commissioners can sometimes struggle when setting these – the aim is to use fair but effective values. I have found the process to be largely built on negotiation. You need to work towards a stretching but realistic target – for example, a target that encourages good practice and for which non-achievement indicates a risk to outcomes or experience. Baselines can help with setting realistic targets as they indicate what is usual for a provider. If the baseline is already good, then the baseline sets the precedent. If the baseline is poor, then a trajectory of targets may be required as a provider improves. If a baseline is not available, then it is common practice to split an annual term into phases, with the first few devoted to developing a baseline while in subsequent phases this baseline is examined and a target negotiated. For example:

- quarter one – provider readiness for baseline collection;
- quarters two and three – provider collects baseline data;
- quarter four – provider and commissioner assess baseline and agree a stretching target for the remaining and subsequent year.

If events conspire against providers – a world-wide pandemic, for instance – ensure you have flexibility to abandon or reassess targets.

Other contributors to outcomes

There can be variation in outcomes due to many factors outside of the control of commissioners and providers. These are always worthy of inspection, especially where a service is benchmarked against other services in different localities. Some of the common causes of variation include:

- structural and process variations – such as staffing mix or availability of equipment for investigations;
- patient characteristics – such as other co-morbidities, their socioeconomic status, cultural differences;
- external factors and accessibility – such as availability and quality of community care services, rurality, availability of hospices;
- environmental factors – such as quality of housing, air quality, climate effects, a pandemic;
- measurement challenges – such as availability of data systems, counting and coding differences, methods of analysis;
- statistical factors – such as random variation and/or statistical anomalies due to small populations.

Being aware of these factors is important. They can never be completely removed, aside from in strict medical trial conditions. Therefore, commissioners need to aware of them but still examine trends that could be indicators of change.

Designing evaluation

Design of evaluation will vary from service to service. It depends on the size and scale of the service, the level of political will or governance it attracts, and the aim of the improvement initiative or service. A large service that needs to meet national standards for safety and quality requires a wide range of indicators, whereas a small service with only local accountability and very limited clinical risk can be evaluated with a few indicators. A common framework approach is helpful for commissioners, as they can use this to adapt their evaluation approach for each project, with proportionality.

When to evaluate

It is particularly important to evaluate when:

- there has been significant investment of resource, such as time or money;
- there is a risk to patient safety;
- it is an innovative or untested approach;
- the subject in question is highly political, a high national or local priority, or very sensitive, with a reputation risk;
- there is a gap in knowledge about how to address a problem.

It can take time and resources to do evaluation on a large scale, so its use should be targeted, with light touch approaches where the criteria mentioned here do not warrant full scrutiny.

Benefits realisation

Benefits realisation is an example of a framework approach to evaluating health and wellbeing. It is the process of identifying positive consequences of change. It has been defined as 'the identification, definition, tracking, realisation, and optimisation of benefits. Benefits management is undertaken throughout the project lifecycle and into operations/ business-as-usual' (Infrastructure and Projects Authority, 2017). My interpretation of the process is shown in Figure 8.1.

The benefits realisation process has greatest impact when implemented right at the outset of identifying need and then throughout the design stages. That said, it can be implemented at any stage, and works for long-standing incumbent services. The process is a simple one. This is outlined in Table 8.2.

Using benefits realisation as a framework for assessing impact of change is a positive stance to take with partners. The following points are key to a successful joint benefits realisation process.

- A shared vision with anticipated outcomes will be useful for all stages – design, implementation, and following delivery. Agreeing what and how you will measure benefits in advance provides clarity.

Figure 8.1: Benefits realisation process

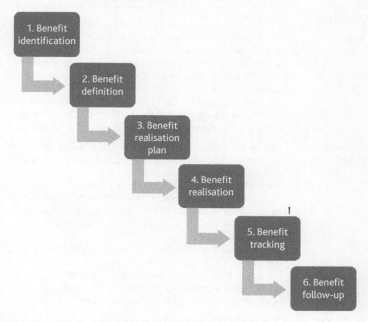

- Start with the patient. Individual and population benefits are key. Financial benefits should not be the driver.
- Identifying system value is important – this is inclusive of financial, social, economic, and community value that is system-wide. Addressing and recognising the system-wide value benefits is a strength of an integrated care system approach.
- Good governance structures ensure that controls and structures are in place to support identification of what will be measured, why, and how. An objective oversight, which ensures matching of outcomes to strategic priorities, adds weight and support to the development of an evaluation process.
- Effective evaluation is dependent on more than just data collection systems and contracts; the culture is important. Acceptance of why change is in place and being measured is essential. Clinical leaders and professional and supporting teams need to clearly understand and support 'why' the change is important. This will support compliance and improve not only the evaluation but also the achievement of outcomes.

Table 8.2: Benefits realisation process

Process step	Key actions
1 Benefit identification	Identify the potential and expected benefits from the initiative. These can be very wide-ranging. Include health and wellbeing outcomes for people, structural and process benefits for providers, financial elements, safety, social impacts, and so on. All potential benefits should be captured, but a process of identifying key benefits can be useful for clarity and focus. These should align with the 'vision' discussed in Chapter 5.
2. Benefit definition	Once you have identified your potential benefits, you need to clearly define what these benefits will look like in practice and how you will evidence them. For example, an identified benefit is that a patient has increased choice and control. This is evidenced as an increase in positive patient-reported experience and an uptake in personalised care and support plans and shared decision-making conversations. If resources are limited, then only the key benefits will be defined with evidence markers. Choose SMART (specific, measurable, achievable, relevant, and timely) benefit indicators where possible, though qualitative evidence is often very persuasive.

3. Benefit realisation plan	The benefits (especially those identified as key) will each have a plan of action covering:
	• their realisation – what needs to be done to achieve them – this is part of your service development plan but specifically for benefits you will include:
	  o what will be different;
	  o what the baseline is;
	  o what the forecast is;
	  o what actions are needed;
	• their analysis – what is needed to collect the evidence and analyse it to ensure it is meaningful (who, what, when, and how);
	• target dates for achievement and for analysis.

4. Benefit realisation	This is the stage of action when changes are implemented and mechanisms for aiding evaluation are initiated.
5. Benefit tracking	Without the right data collected at the right time and in the right way, it will be very difficult to analyse benefits. The Healthcare Financial Management Association (2021) share the following useful considerations for identifying metrics: • What is the baseline service? • What is the future input and output change? • What is the future outcome change?

Table 8.2: Benefits realisation process (continued)

Process step	Key actions
	• What does the change mean for the residual original service (if applicable)? • Where will the measures and metrics materialise (it will not always be with the core service provider)? • How will a 'shift' in service delivery be followed by existing resources to improve efficiency? • What data capture systems exist to map financial and non-financial measures? • What further data and information are required to assess whether benefits have been realised?
6. Benefit follow-up	Once you have analysed the benefits achieved, it is time to consider: • further improvements or corrections to the service; • spread and scale, where successful; • how to ensure sustainability of benefits; • sharing benefits for stakeholder confidence.

Improving data collection

The importance of good data collection cannot be understated. Without it, evidence may be poor and the persuasive argument for further improvements in the future may be weakened. Or, in a worse case scenario, the ability to discover impacts that could be harmful or wasteful is lost. The list that follows includes high-level pointers, but I would recommend that data and intelligence for any sizeable project warrants a workstream of its own with experts from all the involved organisations around the table.

For data collection, consider:

• Does everyone involved know what they are recording and then subsequently collecting? Are national definitions and information standards used appropriately? Is training required?
• Is everyone coding and counting the same things? Is an information standard required that clearly defines clinical terms?
• Are data quality processes in place? Snap-shot audits may give assurance (or not) that data collection is good quality.

When it comes to analysis:

- Are there consistent methodologies for analysis, especially where more than one team is involved across a wider footprint? Where possible, use the same data from the same systems, using the same statistical analysis methods, and have analysis done by a single team.
- Consistency of data: How does the current data look compared to the historic picture? Are there unexplained peaks or troughs that need to be investigated?

In terms of timeliness:

- Preferably use real-time data, or as close to this as possible. Historical datasets have their place but when analysing change, it needs to be more responsive.

In terms of support for non-NHS providers:

- Support the use of comparable quality data collection. Is training required or would a VCSE provider, such as a hospice, benefit from integrated care system support to develop IT systems – they won't necessarily have the infrastructure of larger providers.
- If required, use contracts as devices to establish standards of data collection. The data quality and improvement plan (Chapter 6) can be used to set out steps to improvement.

In relation to reducing the burden of data collection:

- Where possible, use data from sources already available.
- Consider the value of each data collection activity – is it worth the time and effort for the information it gives you? Lots of data is good but sometimes you need to prioritise and focus on quality.

Triangulation of data

Analysis of data is discussed in Chapter 4; however, when considering the evaluation of outcomes for some services or interventions, it is worth stressing the importance of triangulating multiple data sources to fully understand the impacts on patients, especially to identify harm or longer-term impacts. Fractured data sources can make spotting harm difficult. For example, if data had been more joined up then it may have been possible to sooner identify the harm caused by the medical device pelvic mesh, which caused women to suffer pain, infection, and other problems, or the harm caused by the epilepsy drug sodium valproate, which can cause birth defects.

Collecting data once and then enabling its frequent use (within information governance rules) by clinicians or others can support appropriate interrogation of data, addressing of clinical questions, and rapid analysis. Commissioners can support this by encouraging curiosity about how a service or change for improvement is working and establishing clinical or organisational ownership of the examination of outcomes, whether they be clinical, social, or environmental.

Unintended consequences

Any evaluation process needs to be open to identifying unintended consequences, whether they be good or bad. Here, an open reporting process incorporated into monitoring arrangements means that providers can share their learning or that stakeholders such as patients or third parties can share their reflections on how a service is received, including unforeseen implications. Even seemingly neutral consequences should be noted.

Evaluation in the commissioning cycle

Evaluation processes are increasingly a joint exercise, with all parties seeking to ensure quality and value with tangible outcomes for people and the population. The new NHS England structures and payment systems certainly aim to support that approach. As examined in Chapter 2, the commissioning cycle involves an ever-evolving process with evaluation the pivotal point for feeding all that is learned into the next round of project development; it also contributes to wider learning in general. Commissioners need to ensure that there are mechanisms in place to feed this learning into future decision making. This is especially true of longer-term outcomes, such as those related to prevention. The ability to discover trends and patterns, draw comparisons, predict future outcomes, and evaluate services builds a stronger system.

Sharing your findings

It is important to share the findings of evaluation. This supports learning and development within your own area, adds to the learning of colleagues in other commissioning areas, allows the public to see that development is taking place, celebrates success, and offers transparency when things need improvement.

Who you intend to share your findings with and within what context will dictate the best format and type of information to use. Information useful for fellow commissioners and organisational stakeholders, including workforce, include:

- data and statistics, which can be used by others to benchmark against;
- case studies, to demonstrate how the development was executed and share key learning points;
- service specifications or local policies employed;
- evaluation criteria and KPIs;
- a summary of any wider social value benefits and plans for longer-term assessment of these.

Information can be made available to the public via:

- local news briefings;
- integrated care system or locality bulletins open to those with an interest;
- social media;
- discussions with public interest groups.

A summary report for large-scale evaluations (and indeed smaller-scale ones where there is valuable learning) is good practice. Not only does it cement for yourself everything you have learned, but it is also a document that can be referred to by others and for future reflection where evaluation is repeated or continuous. Add all key findings in this report, but it is also an excellent vehicle for including discussion on wider social value, which is generally more qualitative than quantitative in nature. I would add any risks that were mitigated, issues that arose, challenges or barriers that remain or were overcome. This would include complaints and summaries of patient or workforce surveys. You can also set out intentions for longer-term monitoring and evaluation.

How to deal with poor performance

When completing evaluation, you may deem an initiative a failure because it hasn't worked in the way you expected it to. If there is evidence to suggest that the provider is the cause of failure, as they haven't been executing the requirements as agreed, then this needs managing. And it can be awkward and difficult to do.

It is worth some investigation as to why this happened. Is it due to lack of understanding (they haven't employed the concept correctly) or buy-in (they don't believe it will work or is the right thing to do) or more practical reasons, such as lack of training or resources? Whatever the reason, there are two key approaches to managing poor provider performance: developmental and punitive. The developmental approach is always preferable to the punitive approach, but commissioners must consider the seriousness of the matter, the risks involved, the legal status, and the current relationship with the provider.

Developmental approach

This starts from the premise that there has been either a mistake along the way of design, miscommunication, or a missed opportunity to share and agree a joint vision. To improve and prevent re-occurrence, a process of development and support can be introduced. First, the provider and commissioner must agree on the reasons for the failure and be clear that these are what will be tackled. Then, a corrective plan will be agreed, with explicit actions for all parties to resolve the issues. It is helpful here for commissioners to take some role in the actions (even if they feel only the provider is at fault) to foster a sense of shared collaboration. It is also helpful to agree what will happen if there is not a successful resolution. This may be the punitive response or cessation of the contract. This brings to the forefront of people's minds what is at stake and reinstates the importance of improvement. If the provider fails to cooperate or does not meet the agreed actions of the performance plan, then punitive action may be the only course.

Punitive approach

The basis of this approach is that although good relationships and partnership working are a key aim, at the end of the day all should work towards improving lives for people and the population using valuable taxpayer money – if this is not happening, then it must be appropriately managed.

As discussed in Chapter 6, levers can be applied, such as financial penalties, restrictions to business, suspension of the contract, and cessation of the contract. This is last resort action and should only be done when there is no other avenue left for collaborative working. If developmental approaches are not implemented first, then commissioners are in danger of ending arrangements that are costly to replace, creating gaps in care and support for their patients, and potentially creating risks of harm.

Evaluating yourself as a commissioner

When completing evaluation of a change project or programme, bear in mind that also on the table for analysis is yourself and your organisation's commissioning practices. Accountability for tangible results is the burden that commissioners bear. There are a few things to consider and perhaps build into a framework of evaluation for all key projects:

- What commissioning resources, including people, were utilised in commissioning? Was this proportionate to the achieved outcomes?
- What quality of effort was deployed? Were the right levels of expertise employed? Was senior oversight at the appropriate level?
- Were the right stakeholders involved and informed? Was the initiative co-produced, and if so, what were the benefits and challenges?
- Did the process incorporate wider strategic aims such as diversity and inclusion, tackling inequalities or climate change?

Invite feedback on the process from key stakeholders to find out if they have views on how you could have completed the process differently.

Although commissioners are busy and may be juggling several other projects, it is worthwhile spending some time reflecting on the process. One option is to have a few hours with the core team and/or partners with time for reflecting, sharing learning, and seeking opportunities to use that learning in the future.

REFLECTIONS FOR LEADERS

Strategic evaluation

Evaluation of the integrated care system can be an important contributor to system development. Good evaluation of strategies employed and processes undertaken can inform executive teams as to how they are performing. Evaluation with a wide focus can support the maturation and growth of an integrated care system. NHS England continues to develop and offer various ways of evaluating system performance and maturity.

Furthermore, evaluation can be evidence of strategy success – that is, confirming you have chosen priorities effectively and are reaping the benefits. Sharing positive evaluation builds trust and confidence in the processes of commissioning. Likewise, where things have not gone to plan, sharing your plans for improvement with transparency will also build a sense of a community, working towards improvement and learning along the way.

Suggestions for success

Where appropriate, avoid a narrow focus when evaluating services or change. It can be tempting to reduce the administrative burden on both providers and commissioners and go for very few metrics – this may be appropriate for small services, but for large-scale initiatives a carefully selected and wide-ranging framework of evaluation metrics will give a fuller picture of impact and will in the long term support improvement initiatives as the benefits are realised.

Use your evaluation findings for not only the service in question, but also to inform future developments. Take the learning and apply it across the process of commissioning both locally and wherever there is opportunity with your regional and national colleagues. It is a common mistake for commissioners to conclude that they haven't done anything specifically new or exciting, but I can say with experience that fellow commissioners are always interested in what you have done and what the outcome was.

9

Health inequalities

Aim

This chapter discusses the importance of identifying avoidable health inequalities and methods of addressing them. This is increasingly a focus for strategy and policy at local and national levels, and rightly so. Understanding how inequalities can affect access to services and good health and wellbeing is crucial in a bid to reduce them and ensure good care is available to all.

Understanding health inequalities

Equality versus equity

Before I delve into commissioning for health inequalities, it is worth spending a few moments on the meaning of equality and equity. There is a distinct difference, and although the term **health inequalities** is routinely used, it is **inequity** between groups that is the issue.

The image in Figure 9.1 is a common one, and it does an excellent job of illustrating the differences between equality and equity. It shows that although we can treat people the same and offer them the same opportunities and access, due to multiple reasons, this is not equity. Some people need additional support to access the same opportunities or offers of care. This means that distribution of resources is required in a way that is not always equal, but offers equity, to take account of need. It is helpful to remember this approach as we consider health inequalities.

Figure 9.1: Equality and equity comparison

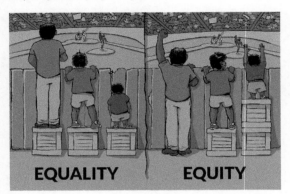

Source: Jayatilleke (2020) Open Government Licence v3.0

What are health inequalities?

The King's Fund define health inequalities as 'avoidable, unfair and systematic differences in health between different groups of people' (Williams et al, 2022). Health inequalities arise for a variety of reasons, including age, sex, race, and religion, but also where we live, where we work, and how financially well off we are. Three key factors that have an impact on health equity are discussed next.

Socioeconomic and deprivation factors

One of the largest impacts on health outcomes is level of deprivation – that is, lack of the material benefits considered to be of basic necessity in society. Figure 9.2, taken from the NHS Long Term Plan, demonstrates the impact that deprivation can have on mortality. Those in the lowest deprivation decile have a lower life expectation by nearly ten years compared to those in the least deprived decile. That is approximately one eighth of a life. Deprivation can encapsulate income, employment, education, health, crime, housing, and the living environment. These are wider determinants of health, meaning they have an impact on our future health, healthcare access, experience, and outcomes. None of these can be considered in isolation, as they have a compound

Figure 9.2: Effect of deprivation on mortality

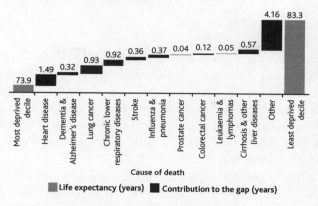

Source: NHS England (2019c) Open Government Licence v3.0

effect. For example, level of education affects employment opportunities, which affects quality of housing, and so on. Or, where a person lives geographically affects access to green spaces and recreation, where they can shop, and what foods they can buy easily, which has an effect on diet.

Table 9.1, adapted from the Healthcare Financial Management Association (2023) briefing *Health inequalities: establishing the case for change*, provides examples of some of these factors and their effects.

Special characteristics

Protected characteristics are personal characteristics protected by law. Under the Equality Act 2010, people are not allowed to discriminate, harass, or victimise another person because of their protected characteristics. That is, you cannot be discriminated against due to your:

- age;
- disability;
- gender reassignment status;
- marriage and civil partnership status;
- pregnancy and maternity status;
- race;

- religion or belief;
- sex;
- sexual orientation.

These characteristics are particularly important to those designing and delivering health and wellbeing provision, because they can contribute to health. For example, women spend a greater proportion of their lives in ill health than men do (Department of Health and Social Care, 2022b), and people from Black African, African Caribbean and South Asian backgrounds are at higher risk of type 2 diabetes (Diabetes UK, 2021).

Inequalities can also arise here due the practicalities or clinical aspects of a characteristic, such as access issues for those who are deaf, or correlations with disease for people from specific

Table 9.1: Wider determinants of health

Determinant	Examples of detriment
Income	• Lack of ability to obtain health-improving goods and healthy foods • Low income is a source of stress • Low income correlates with poor health choices • Low income correlates with poor mental health
Housing	• Increased risk of illness with poor-quality housing and overcrowding • Increased risk of respiratory diseases with poor ventilation • Fuel poverty
Environment	• Lack of access to green spaces for exercise and wellbeing • Exposure to air pollution
Transport	• Increased risk of road accidents in deprived areas • Reduced access to health services, education, and work with limited access transportation due to cost or availability
Education	• Correlation of shorter life expectancy with lower levels of education
Work	• Correlation of lower life expectancy with unemployment • Increased exposure to work-related hazards • Stress associated with poorer job security
Geography	• Reduced availability of services in rural areas and the associated travel costs of attending rural premises

backgrounds. And they can also arise from prejudice and discrimination. Behaviours of workforce or people designing services can further disadvantage people either advertently or inadvertently through unconscious bias or ignorance.

Socially excluded groups

These groups include people who are homeless, those with substance dependencies, travelling communities, and those in the justice system. These people may not be contactable by phone or post, they generally do not proactively seek care, and they are inadvertently denied access to healthcare.

Access

Access to services, care, and support can be affected in multiple ways. Physical access is the first thing that comes to mind. Can people reach and enter the physical premises of the care and support they need? Commissioners can examine these physical access needs. Mobility issues can be easily addressed. This may include physical changes to premises, such as the addition of ramps or lifts. Working with local partners, transport access can be improved to meet people's needs – extra buses to hospitals or shuttles from certain communities might be provided. It is also important to consider reducing barriers that might be off-putting to those who need to attend a service. Is the signage clear and in the right place? Is it in the right language? Where care is provided in the home, can the home be made safe for the workforce to provide care? Considering the physical access needs is an important step in service design.

Another barrier to access is information. Do people have the right information at the right time and in the right format for them to access the care and support they need? Making sure that information is accessible and that it is provided in appropriate formats is a key part of making sure that everyone can understand and therefore benefit from what is provided. First and foremost, do people have the right information to make an informed decision about whether a service is right for them? Are advocates for services in place for communities? Is information provided in languages to meet the needs of the ethnic minority populations? Some language used in health and social care settings can be problematic, because it may involve jargon or acronyms that are not known to all. Getting the language right so that everyone understands each other is essential. Once in a service, are interpreters or people who can use sign language available? Commissioners need to understand their community needs and be ready to support them.

Another barrier to access is lack of support or the right conditions to promote attendance or use. For example, socially excluded groups, busy working people in low-income areas, and even young people sometimes need service access shaped to their needs. There are approaches that can tackle the restrictions facing these groups – for example, a homeless person can receive wound care on the street, a person who cannot take time of work may benefit from screening in the workplace, and a young person struggling to control their insulin levels may find that peer groups are a more welcoming place to learn self-management.

Current challenges for health inequalities

COVID-19

The COVID-19 pandemic shone an unfavourable light on the impact of health inequalities for people. The pandemic exacerbated the impact on people who are affected by the factors that contribute to inequalities. I discuss the impact and the learning from the pandemic further in Chapter 11, but it is a positive note that the pandemic has highlighted this priority and that national policy has been developed for tackling avoidable health inequalities.

Cost of living crisis

From 2021 to the time of writing in 2024, we are amid a cost-of-living crisis. Households in the UK have experienced a significant fall in living standards due to multiple factors, including the lasting impact of the pandemic and increasing fuel and food prices. This has had an impact on people's health, as socioeconomic inequalities have worsened. For example, severity of ill health has worsened, mental health has declined, and people are increasingly unable to attend appointments, fund recreation or health improvements, keep their homes heated, or provide themselves and their families with a good diet (Finch, 2022).

The impact of this crisis will be with us for some time with increased pressures on public services and voluntary, community and social enterprise (VCSE) organisations. As integrated care systems plan long-term strategies, they need to factor in this challenge.

Why do health inequalities matter?

Obviously, health inequalities matter to people and their families. Putting the greater incidence of ill health and slower recovery aside, the limited or barrier-ridden access to care and support must be frustrating, isolating, and stressful. But these inequalities also matter to those planning and delivering health and wellbeing services. Not least because of the morality of the lack of fairness and the lost ability to reduce harm, but because inequalities create demand, more ill health, and increased financial pressure.

Today there is a clear national requirement for tackling this unwarranted variation. This and the other reasons discussed in this section make health inequalities a clear priority for commissioners.

Financial drivers

In 2016, researchers at the University of York calculated that socioeconomic inequalities cost the NHS £4.8 billion per year (Asaria et al, 2016). Their research suggests that in the most deprived fifth of neighbourhoods (compared to the most affluent fifth), there was 72 per cent more emergency admissions and 20 per cent more planned admissions. This research is one of many studies that show similar findings. Other unnecessary costs include:

- missed appointments due to work or transport issues;
- emergency care due to lack of prevention;
- inappropriate usage, such as attending Accident and Emergency as primary care was not accessible in working hours;

- exacerbation of ill health or slowed recovery due to living conditions or stress.

And this impact is in relation to health alone; the wider costs to wider society are much higher.

Policy drivers

Policy for inequality has been around for a while, with duties under the Equality Act 2010 and its public sector equality duty. These seek to ensure that public bodies take equality considerations into account when exercising their functions and making decisions.

The Health and Social Care Act 2012 tightened up the legal requirements for the NHS's responsibility to tackle health inequalities. The is set out as: 'Exercising functions in relation to the health service, the Secretary of State must have regard to the need to reduce inequalities between the people of England with respect to the benefits that they can obtain from the health service.'

The Health and Care Act 2022 strengthened the legal duty and obligation for organisations and included the duty to address inequalities regarding access and outcomes. Furthermore, following the updated 2022 Act, integrated care boards now face a new annual assessment of their duties to reduce inequalities. This includes the need to share at least one equality objective which is specific and measurable. This assessment requirement helps keep the legal duty foremost in the minds of system leaders.

Good to know: Institutional racism

Macpherson (1999) notes that

> Institutional racism is the collective failure of an organisation to provide an appropriate and professional service to people because of their colour, culture, or ethnic origin. It can be seen or detected in processes, attitudes and behaviour which amount to discrimination through unwitting prejudice, ignorance, thoughtlessness, and racist stereotyping, which disadvantage minority ethnic people.

This definition was offered following the Macpherson inquiry into the Stephen Lawrence murder. In response to this case, and others like it, NHS bodies now have several policy documents and guidance on issues of cultural sensitivity and eradicating institutional racism.

These guides and policies are helpful, but it does require more to make a real change. It is everybody's job to tackle racism. It is simply not enough to be 'not racist'; those working in public services need to be 'anti-racist'. The two terms may seem equal, but a person who is anti-racist will speak up and say that a behaviour is not acceptable. This doesn't have to be done in an antagonistic way, but you can clearly signal that you don't accept racism. John Amaechi has shared a video explaining this concept for those who wish to understand it better (see BBC, 2020). These small acts will be cumulative, and they support a move towards tackling racism in the workplace.

Addressing health inequalities

Inequity in society is not something that integrated care systems can eradicate (though they can certainly contribute to reducing it). Therefore, what is the key objective of health and social care bodies for tackling health inequalities? A useful comment is offered by Whitehead (1991): 'Equity in health implies that ideally everyone should have a fair opportunity to attain their full health potential and, more pragmatically, that no one should be disadvantaged from achieving this potential, if it can be avoided.' I believe that this suggests that the aim is not to eradicate all health differences, but to remove or reduce those that result from factors considered avoidable or unfair. This is why you will often see the phrase 'avoidable' or 'unwarranted' health inequalities. It is these inequalities that are in the gift of organisational bodies to identify and reduce or remove.

Identifying health inequalities

Before they can attempt to address inequalities, commissioners need to understand where these exist and for whom. Good commissioning models have embedded population health analysis as business as usual and understand the population needs. Good data and effective analysis show where services are not being utilised as expected, and demographic data uncover trends in poor uptake or access for particular groups. In addition to local data, there are sources of national data. These are helpful for comparisons with areas with similar demographics. One of the key sources is the Office for National Statistics. They offer a dataset with patterns and trends of ill health and death by measures of socioeconomic status. Commissioners can also use the datasets specific to each of the protected characteristics that are held by a variety of national bodies. NHS England offers a national health inequalities dashboard that is currently open to public sector organisations. The dashboard combines data from numerous sources to aid integrated care systems as they identify local inequality priorities.

Other sources of information include complaints, workforce concerns, patient surveys, and feedback from external patient groups, like Healthwatch. These sources are more likely to indicate that which is harder to measure, such as prejudice and discrimination due to protected characteristics. Through triangulation of these sources, behaviours and processes that are not in keeping with equity can be identified.

Understanding the local context is another step to take. This is where co-production, if done effectively, can highlight what is missing, where, for whom, and why. I examine co-production in Chapter 5, but it is worth reiterating its importance in the context of addressing inequalities. The very act of trying to understand people's needs and concerns is a step towards reducing inequity.

Examining differences between groups and their health and social care needs is obvious, but don't overlook people's basic rights too. For example, people have a basic right to freedom, inclusion, choice, and ordinary things like friendships, employment, and being part of a community. How can services contribute to those rights for people with learning disabilities or the socially excluded? Also, remember when working with these groups that people are not just one characteristic – they have a variety of needs and preferences and may have more than one inequity, challenging their access and outcomes for health and wellbeing.

Creating conditions for change

In 2022, NHS England in partnership with The Health Foundation and the Yorkshire and Humber Academic Health Science Network, developed a guide for action on health inequalities (NHS England, 2022b). They acknowledged that there is no single solution for tackling inequalities, but they did share common ingredients for success. These are adapted as follows:

- Creating an enabling system context, including:
  - o enabling strong all-system approaches with visible collaboration with wider partners;
  - o dedicating a senior responsible officer to tackling inequalities;
  - o recognising and rewarding efforts;
  - o ensuring good data and intelligence that is system-wide and supported by information-sharing agreements;
  - o implementing governance, structures, and frameworks that incorporate the investigation and inclusion of tackling inequalities in all stages of design and development;
- Building clear and shared understanding, including:
  - o ensuring all datasets include the key data for examination and that this is recorded accurately and in a timely manner;
  - o creating a shared and stretching vision;
  - o testing data with voices of lived experience;
  - o co-producing solutions and involve communities;
- Maintaining a sense of urgency and commitment to act, including:
  - o raising awareness and stressing the importance of tackling inequalities;
  - o seeking board-level endorsement;
  - o engaging hearts and minds by stressing why this matters to the local population and its people;
  - o committing resources, such as financial resources, people, expertise, and premises;
  - o stressing the legal duties and statutory responsibilities;
- Focusing on implementation, impact, and evaluation, including:
  - o developing meaningful and specific action plans with clear milestones;

o building on successes with use of learning from small to big scale;
o developing frameworks to assess equity in initiatives and their evaluation;
o promoting innovation and disruption to the status quo – being brave and taking risks;
o promoting and communicating plans and actions;
o establishing a common brand for the work on inequity and building trust in the brand within the community.

And I would add:

• Endurance:
o developing long-term planning cycles that exceed political attention spans and leadership tenure with ambitions built to last.

Many of these good practice actions can be scaled down for small-scale initiatives. For example, a small group of organisations may agree a charter, with partners signing up to achievable commitments, they can use local intelligence to identify inequity, and they can co-produce on a small scale and showcase their successes throughout the neighbourhood or wider area.

Core20PLUS5

Core20PLUS5 (see Figure 9.3) is a national framework launched in 2021 following the pandemic. It aims to support commissioners to reduce healthcare inequalities for people of all ages by directing action where it is most needed. It takes a multifaceted approach of identifying key inequalities to guide integrated care systems. The make-up of the framework for adults and children is summarised in Table 9.2.

Applying Core20PLUS5

Integrated care systems are expected to know their Core20PLUS5 population, including their needs. These identified groups will then form the basis of local priorities and initiatives for tackling health inequalities and improving quality.

NHS England has supported the use of this framework in several ways. There has been funding available to pump-prime

Figure 9.3: The Core20PLUS5 model for adults

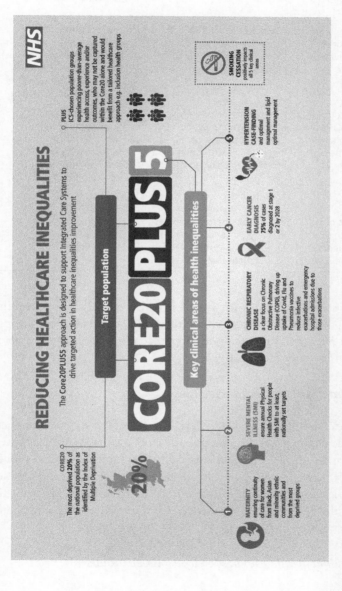

Table 9.2: The Core20PLUS5 framework

Element of model	Adults	Children and young people
Core20 National deprivation	The most deprived 20% of the national population as identified by the national Index of Multiple Deprivation.	The most deprived 20% of the national population as identified by the national Index of Multiple Deprivation plus wider sources of data, such as national child mortality data.
PLUS Local deprived population groups	Populations include ethnic minority groups, people with learning disability, people with long-term health conditions, and socially excluded groups.	Populations may include ethnic minority groups, children with autism, young carers, looked-after children, and children in socially excluded groups.
5 Five clinical areas of focus which require accelerated improvement	1. Maternity 2. Severe mental illness 3. Chronic respiratory disease 4. Early cancer diagnosis 5. Hypertension case-finding and management	1. Asthma 2. Diabetes 3. Epilepsy 4. Oral health 5. Mental health

the scheme along with national and regional commissioning support. Quality improvement methodologies have been shared, and networks have been developed across systems in support of the movement for change.

Examples of tackling inequalities

The case studies in Table 9.3 are a sample of locally based projects undertaken to tackle inequalities. These have been adapted from the NHS England inequality resources and case studies (NHS England, 2024f) and their guide to tackling inequalities (NHS England, 2022b), which are both worth reading in full for the learning on approaches for addressing inequalities and overcoming challenges.

Tackling inequalities in socially excluded groups

As discussed previously, co-production is an effective way to ensure that approaches for tackling inequalities are designed to be

Table 9.3: Case studies for tackling inequalities

Inequity	Key actions
Vaccination uptake by different groups	The bottom 10% according to the Index of Multiple Deprivation were targeted; this comprised ethnic minorities and White working-class communities living in poverty. Actions: • dedicated community engagement role; • promotion through social networks and community organisations; • co-produced approach with VCSE staff; • part-funded health coaching roles for conversations with patients; • pop-up vaccination clinics.
Health and wellbeing of people at risk of heart failure	People living in the highest deprivation quintile were targeted. Actions: • action learning sets with professionals to link local data and design, explore models of care, and track and monitor interventions; • menu of local support offered, including social prescribing appointments, medicine reviews, annual health checks, links to peer support.
Physical checks for people with severe mental illness	People with severe mental illness were targeted. Actions: • health care assistants recruited to perform annual physical health checks; • proactive outreach into the community with point of care testing machines; • collaboration with mental health trust providers to coordinate care; • collaboration with VCSE for follow-up support.
Cancer screening uptake	Ethnic minority groups were targeted. Actions: • behaviour science approach using nudge interventions (Thaler and Sunstein, 2008) and messaging to individuals – nudge intervention theory is that the offer does not alter but people are supported and 'nudged' to make better decisions for themselves; • nudge interventions designed with VCSE organisations, public health and screening teams.
Oral healthcare	Socially excluded groups, children who are looked after, and vulnerable migrants were targeted. Actions: • homeless-friendly dental practices (developed following work with homeless charities) offering dedicated sessions;

(continued)

Table 9.3: Case studies for tackling inequalities (continued)

Inequity	Key actions
	• local charities supported to book people in and support them to attend; • single pathway for children who are looked after, with standardised assessment forms; • carers given advice and guidance on oral care; • screening questionnaire developed in appropriate languages; • referral to foundation training, with costs covered.
Medical information on prescription bottles	Ethnic and linguistically diverse groups were targeted. Actions: • a new service providing bilingual dispensing labels in patient's language of choice.
Health and wellbeing of fishermen who are unable to attend regular health services	Fishermen and their families were targeted as they struggle to plan time for regular healthcare. Actions: • NHS health checks in mobile health events; • access to mental health support; • taking care to the quayside – delivered and adapted to the local environment; • building rapport and trust with the community.

effective. However, some groups may be more difficult to involve in co-production in a meaningful way, such as socially excluded people, but that should not be a reason to not try. Dr Nigel Hewitt (2018) suggests some methods of involving and improving outcomes for these groups:

- Excluded groups should be prioritised to reflect the intensity of their needs and exceptionally poor outcomes.
- Personalisation of people's needs is key – avoid a one-size-fits-all approach based on assumptions.
- De-institutionalisation should be prioritised. Where possible, allow people the option of staying in ordinary housing rather than hostels or refuges that congregate people.
- A 'housing first' policy can employ system-wide approaches to provide prompt housing and integrate physical health, mental health, and addictions support in an integrated and coordinated package.
- Deliver interventions in the community and on the streets.

- Values-driven care, which promotes trust, fairness, respect, and equality, is important.

These are new ways of working for many areas, but the cohesion of health, social care, housing, justice, and the VCSE sector can open doors for effective responses where the commissioning for these groups can be taken off the 'too hard' pile.

Harnessing prevention opportunities

There are multiple approaches for preventing ill health, and this section includes only a few examples that aim to reduce inequalities for specific groups. Public Health England are committed to prevention as a means of reducing health inequalities; this is a clearly stated aim throughout their *PHE Strategy 2020–25* (Public Health England, 2019). Their expertise is crucial in this area and close working with public health teams will maximise results related to prevention of health inequalities.

Equity from birth

There is general agreement that children from disadvantaged backgrounds tend to have poorer health and wellbeing later in life. This can be due to multiple factors, such as diet, environment, access to play opportunities, access to peers, and development of social skills and language. The *Bright Futures* report (Local Government Association, 2017) recognises the benefits of a good start in life and sets out priority areas for local authorities to aspire and work towards. Those pertinent to local governments and health are adapted and summarised as follows:

- A stronger focus on outcomes for children:
  - o This recognises that the responsibility for achieving improved outcomes lies not just with one organisation, but with all bodies working together, including collaborations between social care, health, and education organisations. This is especially true for improving the safeguarding response.
  - o Improving outcomes for children and considering families should be a golden thread running through all departments.

For example, the *Bright Futures* report suggests that the biggest difference made to children's lives is the availability of safe and comfortable housing, which is outside the remit of children's services for social care and health. Sharing appropriate information across the local authority and health bodies will enable this focus on improving outcomes for children to become more of a reality.

- Consistently strong local leadership:
  o Strong leadership and governance processes are vital building blocks for improvement. They support an effective focus on priorities and lead the way for collaboration across agencies and suitably reaching ambitions for improvement.
- A culture of continuous improvement:
  o While it is important that services for health and social care are rigorously scrutinised and inspected, these processes should not become barriers to improvement, as it has been recognised that inspections and negative judgements can worsen performance. There is a recommendation that assessment of performance should become more continuous and less disruptive. Continuous improvement should be supported regardless of rating and should be coupled with transparency and openness for those who continually seek improvements and are encouraged to identify and address poorer areas of performance.
- The right support for children at the right time:
  o 'Early help' is now a well-recognised term, and it reflects the importance of supporting families with young children. It is a framework response that supports improved outcomes by improving access to support from multiple agencies at the time of need. The Department for Levelling Up, Housing and Communities and the Department for Education (2022) produced the *Early Help System Guide* and toolkit to help organisations implement effective early help systems.
  o Multiple partners working together for early years is crucial for wraparound support for families who need it. An example of this way of working in action includes the 'team around the child' model. Here, multiple professionals work alongside the family to plan and initiate activities that will support the child and family. The aim is to wrap around

the child and family as an integrated whole, thereby sharing insight, agreeing responsibilities, and reducing duplication.

- Strengthened morale and support for social workers:
  - o The success of children's services is heavily reliant on a skilled workforce, but recruiting and retaining social workers is an issue for many councils. Morale is generally low and public perception of these valuable staff is damaging despite significant improvements in, for example, child homicides. Case load is often a concern and coupled with dwindling local authority funding, this is a difficult issue to tackle. There are some steps councils can take to support social workers, such as good-quality human resources and back office support, as well as providing effective electronic devices, and so on.
  - o Local authorities can make efforts to champion social workers. They can make stories of success, reward efforts, and generally share a picture of positivity for social workers in their area.
- Prevention of ill health:
  - o Public health and health services can contribute to the prevention of ill health in many ways, including vaccinations, oral health services, and messages on healthy eating and tackling obesity. These services and others are offered to the whole population, but by targeting specific groups professionals can contribute to reducing the health gap between those with advantages and those with health inequalities.

Life-long social protection

In addition to support and protection in our early years, we all benefit from life-long social protection. This includes systems for those who require support due to old age, illness, disability, or loss of income, and those who provide unpaid care services to loved ones. This level of support changes with successive governments and the amount of funding and strength of policy commitments for these groups fluctuates over the decades. However, local governments and their system partners can take steps to ensure that these groups do not suffer from inequity of access to services, such as physical and mental health services, and where possible there are multi-agency processes and partnerships to proactively support people with most need.

Here, the advantage of neighbourhood-based systems are advantageous. These groups of local organisations know their population well and can plan and implement support for targeted groups in their area.

Unpaid carers

Unpaid carers are a particular group in need of recognition and support. Due to their caring responsibilities, they are often unable to adequately access health and care support for themselves; their health may suffer because of their care duties, and it can affect employment opportunities. Young carers, those aged 5 to 17 years old, suffer adverse effects of their caring duties well into their adult life due to impacts on their health, education, social growth, and opportunities for employment.

Commissioners can recognise the value of unpaid carers, the impact they have on managing public service burden, and the role they have for coordinating care for their loved one. The King's Fund estimate unpaid carers provide the equivalent of four million paid care workers (Fenney et al, 2023). In return, commissioners need to identify and pay appropriate attention to the diverse needs that unpaid carers have. Actions commissioners can take include:

- Strengthening processes to identify unpaid carers – they cannot be supported if they are invisible. They can be difficult to identify, especially if they do not see themselves as a carer. Services in contact with patients can be encouraged to think about carer arrangements and identify carers. Training and inclusion in processes can support this.
- Offering carers an assessment of their needs, and identifying what matters to them – this personalised assessment can better shape a follow-up offer of support. This support offer may include help with managing their own health and wellbeing, respite care, or access to peer support and wellbeing services.
- Offering flexibility to enable carers to access their own care more easily – access can be more difficult due to their caring

responsibilities, so consider access to clinics outside of usual hours or home visits. Caring responsibilities can have adverse health and wellbeing impacts, which in turn can cause a breakdown in caring ability.

- Embedding identification and support offers as standard into all relevant contracts – monitor and evaluate the success of these actions with carer-reported quality indicators (like a patient-reported outcome measure or a patient-reported experience measure; see Chapter 8).
- Where wanted, offering education, training, and information to upskill and support unpaid carers – this can create a greater feeling of confidence and autonomy to those carers who wish for it, such as parents caring for children.
- Raising the profile of carers – these are vital contributors to the health and care system and should be seen as valued partners. Recognise unpaid carers across the system and include their support needs in partnership approaches such as joint strategic needs assessments.

Training the workforce

Training the workforce in issues of inequality has two key aims. The first is that it aims to upskill the workforce in practical ways to take actions to tackle inequalities, and the second is that it will contribute to change in culture and bring 'hearts and minds' on the journey for lasting and effective change. Staff training can:

- foster a deeper understanding of equality and equity;
- improve understanding of the impact on outcomes and experiences for people, and on demand and cost for systems;
- share how to recognise and reduce inequity;
- share how to reduce and tackle prejudice and discrimination;
- provide clarity on legal responsibilities for the organisation and for individuals;
- educate staff on using equality impact assessments for service change;
- demonstrate how diverse and inclusive teams are more effective.

Training should be universal for all staff, including those who have no contact with patients, and it should be refreshed annually.

Clinical staff should receive additional training appropriate for the people they care for. For example, cancer teams who need to be able to recognise when inequalities can affect a person's ability to complete treatment or may impact on their health and wellbeing. This includes the financial impacts while unable to work, opportunities for accessing support, and cultural and spiritual preferences for those nearing end of life.

Good to know: Equality impact assessments

Equality impact assessment is a tool used to examine and identify the impact of decisions, policies, and service changes on people with protected characteristics. It examines risk of inequality – and where there is a risk, highlights the need for it to be considered, removed, or mitigated. This due regard to the impact on inequalities creates a conscious consideration by those examining the change in question, whether it be for strategic or operational reasons. The final assessment document can also be shared for transparency of due consideration and any action taken.

This tool takes the reviewer through a series of questions, prompting them to consider each characteristic individually in relation to the proposed change. Where there are no identified impacts, the activity can proceed. If there are identified risks, those leading the activity can adapt or change the action, stop the action, or proceed with caution where there are no other options available or risks cannot be mitigated further. In these cases, close review is required at frequent intervals and the risk should be included on risk registers.

I would recommend using these as a sense-check tool right at the outset of any policy or service design, and repeated in the stages of design and then once more with the final product. It will help keep you focused on potential impacts. Generally, once established, an annual review is recommended.

A diverse workforce

Diversity and equality in the workforce are important factors for designing and delivering quality services. There are two key reasons for this. First, a diverse workforce can contribute to identifying, designing, and delivering actions to tackle inequity, which can result in reduced health inequalities. Second, a workforce that is not diverse can lead to decreased motivation and productivity, less engagement, and increased turnover of staff (Sarter and Cookingham Bailey, 2023). These features impact on the services delivered and the outcomes for people.

This requirement for diverse teams relates to those delivering care but also those commissioning it. A room full of people who all look and think the same and have the same experiences will struggle to come up with new solutions or be able to think outside of the box they have created for themselves.

Good care is not possible without the critical contribution of a broad range of people, covering different genders, ethnicities, disabilities, religions, national origins, sexual orientations, ages, and other characteristics. Several studies demonstrate improved quality of care for patients, a more sustainable workforce supply, and increased efficiency of services (Gomez and Bernet, 2019; NHS England, 2023d).

There are specific conditions that can contribute to the development of a diverse and inclusive workforce. These relate to:

- Data:
  - o Collate sufficient information and data to enable a more nuanced understanding of the challenges that staff experience, including within and across specific groups. This can include protected characteristics and socioeconomic background.
  - o This demographic data can be analysed alongside recruitment, experience of work, progression, and retention of workforce.
  - o A standardised approach for all system organisations can be rolled out to achieve consistency of reporting on workforce and support benchmarking.
- Evidence-based approaches:
  - o Implement evidence-based approaches to address specific challenges.
  - o Include cultural awareness in staff training.
  - o Review job descriptions for cultural barriers.
  - o Ensure jobs are advertised throughout communities to invite applications form the wider population.

- Resources and responsibilities:
  - o Confirm a budget that is ring-fenced for improving diversity of the workforce.
  - o Have equality and diversity leaders in place at integrated care board level and for each employer – accountability and responsibilities will be clear.
  - o Support staff networks.

REFLECTIONS FOR LEADERS

Racism and diversity

Although there are many policies and guides available for handling racism and diversity problems, it will take courage to truly tackle these issues. Large strides have been made but it is very much a work in progress. There is often an urge to cover up or minimise racist or discriminatory events, and leaders can be hesitant to act.

Today's leaders need to be bold and courageous. They need to recognise when something is not right and do the right thing for the right reasons. Now is the time to be creative with solutions and build momentum for change. Leaders can be role models for change and take their organisation and community along with them.

Suggestions for success

It can seem daunting to consider inequalities and design effective solutions to tackle them. My advice would be to start small and take multiple steps in identifying them and reducing their impact. These incremental steps will have a cumulative effect and will offer you a wealth of learning.

Your allies here are people with voices of lived experience and those working and living in local communities. They will be invaluable on the journey to improvement. Resources and time spent on co-producing change are good investments.

10

Personalised care

Aim

Personalised care approaches aim to ensure that care is tailored to the person and that they have choice and control where it is appropriate. Incorporating these approaches throughout the design of services for health and care will improve outcomes and experiences for people. This chapter describes the six components of the comprehensive model for personalised care, how to apply them, and how they can help improve outcomes for people.

What is personalised care?

Personalised care aims to provide people with the power, and the right conditions, to make choice and control achievable and meaningful. It means people are actively involved in the way their care is planned and delivered, based on 'what matters' to them and their individual strengths, cultural needs, and preferences. This happens within a system that supports people to stay well for longer and makes the most of the expertise, capacity, and potential of people, families, and communities in delivering better health, access, wellbeing, outcomes and experiences.

Personalised care is a business-as-usual requirement in the NHS Long Term Plan (NHS England, 2019c) and therefore is an important consideration for providers and commissioners as they deliver, design, and contract services for the future. NHS England policy suggests that personalised care is central to a new service model for the NHS, including within integrated care systems. The aim is that people have a more diverse range of options, better support, and properly joined-up care at the right time and in the optimal care setting. This approach and the six components make up the comprehensive model of personalised care (NHS England, 2019d). The components are:

1. Shared decision making.
2. Personalised care and support planning.
3. Enabling choice, including legal rights to choice.
4. Social prescribing and community-based support.
5. Supported self-management.
6. Personal health budgets and integrated personal budgets.

The comprehensive model guidance (NHS England, 2019d) suggests that the six components need to be delivered together and in full for the maximum benefit. Although I would agree with this approach, it is sometimes more realistic to incorporate the elements in stages, building confidence in the processes until a full model is reached for the particular care condition to be improved. Or it may be that only some of the components will lend themselves well to the area being developed. The model was first introduced in 2019 and so many health and care systems will now be familiar with the components and have some experience and expertise in their application. Spreading and scaling the approaches is now the aim of many.

The benefits of personalised care

It is a generally agreed concept that where people have greater choice and control for their physical and mental health, there are potential benefits in outcomes and experience. The supported choice and control offered to people can also play a part in reducing health inequalities as the approach recognises and encompasses individual needs.

NHS England guidance suggests there are positive impacts from personalised care on patients, their families, professionals, and the wider system (NHS England, 2019d). The potential benefits include:

- better outcomes for patients and their families – people report feeling more in control and happier with their care. They feel enabled to make decisions for themselves alongside professionals. Outcomes can be improved as care and support is tailored to them;
- reduced inequalities – due to the removal of barriers with the introduction of improved personal choice, people's needs are more closely met;
- stronger communities – they build resilience and actively support their residents;
- improved patient/professional relationship – the cultural divide between patient and professional is eroded as the balance is restored to a partnership;
- integration between professional groups – as people live longer there are more people living with more than one complex condition. Personalised approaches can dissolve some of the silo working and join up clinical teams for a single approach;
- integration between providers – personalised care approaches promote and support interagency working as personalised plans are shared;
- financial savings – although people living longer evokes images of extra demand, many stay well for longer and manage their own conditions better, which reduces demand in unplanned care, reliance on healthcare professionals, and fewer exacerbations or slower deterioration of conditions;
- integrated care system duties – integrated care systems can demonstrate they are meeting the commitments in the NHS Long Term Plan, providing legal rights for choice and personal health budgets, and taking steps to reduce inequalities.

The elements of personalised care

Shared decision making

Shared decision making is a process which allows a patient to be involved as they wish in the decision making about their care and treatment. It is a shared partnership between patient and clinician. This may seem like an obvious thing we would all want, but often in traditional healthcare culture, clinicians can make assumptions about people and what is best for them, and make decisions about care without discussing the options fully.

The shared decision making process supports people to understand the diagnosis they have and the options they face. In a process of deliberation, they are supported to talk about what matters to them in terms of their attitude to risk, the trade-offs they are willing to make, and the outcomes that are important to' them. Finally, a decision is made in partnership with their professional team.

To maximise the benefits from shared decision making, people are supported to:

- understand the care, treatment, or options available and all the risks, benefits, and consequences of those options – this may include doing nothing;
- make decisions, based on good evidence-based information, that reflect their personal preferences;
- be as involved as they wish in choosing options.

It is a shared process, with a flow of information between the parties, the aim being to come to the best option for the patient as an individual.

Benefits of shared decision making

Where people are informed and involved in decision making, they are more likely to adhere to treatment plans, have more realistic expectations, and ultimately have better outcomes and experiences.

A systematic review (Durand et al, 2014) suggests that shared decision making improves outcomes for people who are disadvantaged. This is especially so where people's health literacy – that is, their ability to understand and use information about health decisions – is addressed using specific techniques and tools to ensure people understand their decisions.

Implementing shared decision making

Shared decision making can be implemented for any non-emergency care decision where there is more than one option. This can be in primary, community, mental health, and acute care settings.

Mapping care pathways for key decision points is a good way of identifying where shared decision making can be implemented. This approach is particularly valuable where there are 'high value' decisions that can have a significant impact, where options may be 'preference sensitive' for people with different values, and where there may be trade-offs, such as quality of life versus length of life.

Teams and clinicians require training for the process of sharing information and to optimise helping people to understand their options. This may be a cultural change for some clinicians and there can be resistance to training – this barrier is known as 'unconscious incompetence' as clinicians do not recognise that they will benefit from learning how to apply the new approach. Time for embedding this change in approach shouldn't be underestimated. A training plan and a phased shift over time is usually realistic and allows professionals to build confidence and trust in the process.

People should be made aware of the process and what their role is, and they should be supported to ask questions. This process enables the 'prepared public'. Co-production can be used when designing how people will be supported through the shared decision-making process.

There are validated tools (Elwyn, 2024; Patient ALS Partner, 2024) available to evaluate how well the process is working. Different care settings may find some are more suitable than others.

Appendix 1 shares some recommended wording that can be adapted for service specifications.

Personalised care and support planning

Personalised care and support planning is a conversation in which there is a holistic exploration of a person's health and wellbeing in the context of their whole life and family situation. The aim is to explore what matters to a person to enable them to have a good life and ensure that they receive the support they need to achieve their desired outcomes. Like shared decision making, people are equal partners in the process; plus it recognises people's skills and strengths as part of the process.

Personalised care and support planning can be implemented across all of health and social care. Therefore, multiple plans can be joined up in a single plan that can be accessed by all appropriate professionals. Ideally, these plans are stored electronically and can be accessed for review and amendment by several professionals, and even the patient themselves.

There is no single template for a personalised care and support plan, but NHS England have shared what the essential criteria are and what a good plan and process will include (NHS England, 2024d). The personalised care and support plan:

- has a clear way of capturing and recording conversations, decisions, and agreed outcomes or goals in a way that makes sense to the person;
- is proportionate, flexible, and coordinated to adapt to the person's health condition, situation, and care and support needs;
- includes a description of the person, what matters to them, and all the necessary elements that would make the plan achievable and effective.

The essential criteria for the process are as follows:

1. People are central in developing and agreeing their personalised care and support plan, including deciding who is involved in the process.
2. People have proactive, personalised conversations which focus on what matters to them, paying attention to their needs and their wider health and wellbeing.
3. People agree the health and wellbeing outcomes they want to achieve in partnership with the relevant professionals.
4. Each person has a sharable, personalised care and support plan, which records what matters to them, their outcomes, and how they will be achieved.
5. People are able to formally and informally review their personalised care and support plan.

Benefits of personalised care and support planning

NHS England (2019d) suggest that where people are involved in proactively shaping care options, they are more likely to be supported effectively, and they will be more likely participate in the care put in place for them. This can lead to improved outcomes and experiences as the plan has more meaning for the affected person. They are more likely to adhere to and fully engage with plans. And as a personalised care and support plan is shared across multiple agencies, the person does not have the frustration of telling their story time and time again – it joins up the care to the person rather than the person hopping from service to service with no coordination.

Implementing personalised care and support planning

Personalised care and support planning can be beneficial to anyone and any pathway, but as it can be a lengthy task, it is more commonly used for people with long-term conditions or where there is complexity of care. Here, it should be built into these pathways as standard. Personalised care and support plans are a must for personal health budgets.

Where a change in culture is required, especially where professionals will struggle with the slightly longer and more reflective process, then training and realistic timescales for rolling out change should be agreed. Incentives such as local Commissioning for Quality and Innovation (CQUIN) goals can support this change.

People need to be fully aware of what the personalised care and support planning process is and what it aims to do for them. Without that understanding, there will not be a meaningful conversation and subsequent plan. People need time and support to develop their plan, and to help them do this they need the right information in a way that they can access and understand. A single coordinator is often used to develop plans with people. They will have appropriate training and can build trusting and effective relationships with people.

Data-sharing agreements may be required as the plan is accessed by multiple agencies. Common language and methods of adding or updating information to the plan must be agreed and protocols of good practice are a good idea as these plans may be used by many agencies. The digital storage and sharing of plans can be tricky but most healthcare, systems have processes in place to enable this or have plans to implement the required digital infrastructure.

Evaluation of the consistency of offer and the quality of the process will require collection of quantitative and qualitative data.

This may be onerous in the early stages but can be scaled down where there is effective rollout. I would recommend that as well as counting numbers of plans completed, it is important to count the offer of plans to patients. And where this offer is not taken up, what were the reasons for this? What would support people to develop a plan that is meaningful to them? Plus, to ensure quality of plans, a snapshot audit at intervals – for example, examination of ten plans every three months – can offer some assurance that they are good quality. Finally, it is worth considering the feedback from patients. A survey or focus group can explore if the process was effective for them and if there is anything they would change – then improvements can be co-produced.

Appendix 1 shares some recommended wording that can be adapted for service specifications.

Enabling choice

Choice, and legal rights to choice, are part of the NHS Constitution (Department of Health and Social Care, 2021; see also Appendix 3). These rights are supported and outlined by NHS England. There are a range of choices available to patients in different circumstances. The NHS Choice Framework (Department of Health and Social Care, 2023) sets out the government's commitment to offering patients choice. The areas where patients have choice include:

- choosing a general practitioner (GP) and GP practice;
- choosing where to go for a first appointment as an outpatient;
- asking to change hospital if you have to wait longer than the maximum waiting time;
- choosing who carries out a specialist test;
- choosing maternity services;
- choosing services provided in the community;
- choosing to take part in health research;
- choosing to have a personal health budget;
- choosing healthcare in an European Economic Area.

I won't examine these rights in detail here, but it is worth noting these legal rights to choice – be aware of what patients are entitled to and avoid creating barriers to choice.

Implementing choice for patients

There are enablers of choice that make the process more meaningful for patients. If these are not in place, then choices may not be utilised or poor choices may be made. Figure 10.1 illustrates the three enablers for choice.

First, people need to be aware that they have choice, and professionals need to be aware that people can exercise this right. All ICBs should have information about rights to choice on their web pages. Other approaches to make people aware of their rights to choice include posters in GP clinics or patient groups engaging with people to spread the message. GPs and other referrers need to tell people about their rights to choice where it applies.

Figure 10.1: Enablers for meaningful choice

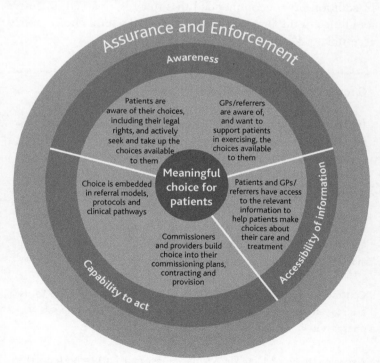

Source: NHS England (2016) Open Government Licence v3.0

Second, people need the right information to be able to make the right choice for them – without this, choice is meaningless. This may include information about waiting times or quality indicators, such as those for safety ratings, effectiveness, and patient experience. This information needs to be in plain English and in a format that is easy to read, and available in other languages as appropriate for the local population. Furthermore, providers need to ensure that their information on the available choice of services is regularly updated, complete and accurate.

Finally, people need to be able to act on their choices. To enable this, commissioners and providers need to embed systems and processes that make choice a reality for people. Systems such as e-Referral should be used as the default option, and monitoring of these should be a priority.

Commissioners need to incorporate the planning of enabled choice into local pathways and service design where it is applicable. In addition, it is recommended that there is a named executive for choice in the integrated care board and a local choice policy accessible to all.

Good to know: NHS e-Referral system

The NHS e-Referral system (e-RS) has been around for some time, and some long-standing commissioners may remember it as Choose and Book. e-RS is a national digital platform that enables electronic patient referrals from a referrer (often a GP) to the provider. It aims to give patients electronic-enabled choice and access within elective services.

e-RS allows patients to choose their first outpatient hospital or clinic appointment – that is, the provider, the day, and the time. This can be done in the GP surgery, online, or on the phone.

Contract changes in 2018 stipulated that NHS providers need to use e-RS for all consultant-led outpatient appointments. Paper referrals were phased out.

A scoping study conducted by Azamar-Alonso et al (2019) concludes that electronic referral systems have the potential to improve the quality of referrals and generally there is high satisfaction with professionals in many settings. The other expected benefits include:

• improved management of referrals between patients and professionals as partners;
• cost and time savings with workflow efficiency;
• fewer missed appointments;
• fewer inappropriate referrals;
• shorter referral to treatment times;
• choice of hospital or specialist;
• choice of appointment date and time;
• improving information on referrals.

(See more at the e-RS web page: https://digital.nhs.uk/services/e-refer ral-service.)

Social prescribing and community-based support

Social prescribing is an approach that connects people with practical, social, or emotional needs to activities, groups, or services in the community. Commonly, the process involves a referral to a social prescribing link worker. This person is skilled in two key areas. First, they can have a conversation with the person about what their needs and preferences are. Together they create a simple personalised care and support plan, which helps the person have choice and control for their own health and wellbeing. Second, the link worker will have a good knowledge and understanding of the community-based support available. They can signpost the person to community support that will be of value to them. Link workers often support the person as they begin the process of utilising this community offer and may even support the person with their first visit or arrange some transport for them to attend.

Link workers often have another very important role in supporting local community-based activities and support offers: they give advice and support to local community group leaders on operating safely, how to apply for grants, and how to support each other as peer groups. Without this support, the community-based support on offer for the scheme would likely reduce, and community resilience would weaken.

Link workers are well placed to see if there are gaps in community-based support. They can support and encourage community groups to meet need in new ways, and they can inform commissioners on gaps. The commissioners can then examine opportunities for strengthening community assets. This identification of gaps is especially important for disadvantaged groups who may have avoidable health inequalities.

Benefits of social prescribing

The expectation is that social prescribing will improve people's wellbeing. It can, if used effectively, provide practical, social, and emotional support, and give some groups of people more control over their lives. Evaluations of local social prescribing schemes generally report reduced pressure on NHS services, reductions in GP consultations, Accident and Emergency attendances, and hospital bed stays. In 2017, the University of Westminster published an evidence summary which identified 28 per cent fewer GP consultations and 24 per cent fewer Accident and Emergency attendances for people receiving social prescribing support (Polley and Pilkington, 2017). This study and others suggest that social prescribing has the potential to improve physical and mental wellbeing. However, more research is needed to establish what works and for whom.

Implementing social prescribing and community-based support

Social prescribing can be offered to any group of people but, as link workers can be inundated with demand, there are often restrictions in place to limit the flow of referrals to those with most need. Priority groups may be people with long-term conditions, low-level mental health issues, the lonely or isolated, and those with complex needs which affect their wellbeing. Most schemes would accept referrals for these priority groups from any referrer, including self-referrals.

National funding is made available to primary care networks for social prescriber link workers, so the majority are employed by primary care, but these roles can be employed by any organisation including those in the VCSE sector. The responsibility of supporting and growing the community-based support sits with the integrated care system. There is considerable developmental support for link workers available through NHS England and the personalised care programme. This programme recognises that these roles require specific training, supervision, and support. The programme supports both the link workers and their employers.

Monitoring of social prescribing processes and uptake is useful as it allows review of:

- demand for support, through numbers of referrals;
- who requires support, using demographic data and conditions;
- uptake of support, by considering whether the people with most need are supported appropriately to access community activities;
- demand for types of support, by looking at what community-based activities people are accessing and where the gaps are;
- effectiveness of support, by examining if people report positive outcomes;
- experience of the link worker, through examining whether they are feeling confident and supported in their role.

Where there is interest in examining health and care system impacts, other data sources can be used, such as historical activity data, which can examine trends in GP appointments, Accident and Emergency attendances, exacerbation of conditions, contacts with community nurses, and so on. This analysis may demonstrate reduced reliance on other services for those groups accessing social prescribing.

Good to know: Compassionate communities

Compassionate communities are naturally occurring sources of kindness, social and emotional support, and compassion for people affected by death, dying, loss and bereavement.

Compassionate communities have two key components. The first are the networks around us. People's closest supportive network will vary, but it might include spouses, children, parents, wider family, and close friends. It can even include neighbours, colleagues, and other people we spend time with. These people will provide caring tasks but also offer us social comfort and friendship. This is our 'inner network'. The 'outer network' comprises of other less well-known friends, people we speak to on a regular basis, perhaps in a shop, and other parents at the school gates. These regular conversations enhance our lives. The inner and outer networks may be from 10 to 200 people, which is a potentially rich resource of support if required.

The second component is made up of the communities we live in. This may be the community we reside in, but it also includes communities we engage with, such as a religious community, a workplace community, and a sports community. These communities provide kindness and compassion through active citizenship.

Compassionate communities are developed naturally, but there are things that can be done to support social movement. These include:

• promoting the value of compassionate communities so people can see how the things they do for others matter;
• building links between interested groups to create supportive networks for growth and support, such as through a compassionate community workshop with information and guidance;
• supporting people who are dealing with death and dying to remain connected socially to others, as social isolation is common during and after loss of a loved one – have clear information on community offers and how to access them;
• aligning NHS and social care services with recognised compassionate community groups, building a culture where the value of compassionate communities is recognised, respected, and understood.

Supported self-management

Supported self-management is an approach to empower people to manage their physical and mental health conditions. This can be achieved in several ways, including:

• peer support – people with similar conditions or health experiences supporting each other with things like understanding of the condition, emotional support, helping recovery, and methods of self-management;

- education – formal education or training to help people develop skills, knowledge, and confidence to manage their own condition safely and effectively;
- health coaching – a less formal form of training that aims to use health coaches in supportive roles to help people reach their own health goals, such as weight loss.

The objective is to upskill people and increase their confidence as an expert on their own health. This includes recognising and managing their symptoms and knowing when and where to get help if needed.

The knowledge, skills, and readiness people need for self-management can be measured. One such measure is the Patient Activation Measure® (PAM®). Assessing individual PAM® levels, or any other equivalent measure can evidence progress made, as you can compare a start position with after a self-management intervention. Knowing a population's or a group's PAM® levels can act as a useful baseline measure, but more importantly it can inform commissioning decisions on how best to support people to achieve effective self-management. Targeted support can be put into place for those who need more support or have low knowledge and skills.

As with all personalised care approaches, best results are achieved when people are focused on 'what matters to them', are equal partners in their health experience, and are supported to form personal health goals in personalised care and support planning. Additionally, there are enhanced success factors when co-producing with voices of lived experience and delivering self-management support with community assets.

Benefits of supported self-management

An independent evaluation (Barker et al, 2017) found that people with high levels of knowledge, skill, and confidence had 19 per cent fewer GP appointments and 38 per cent fewer Accident and Emergency attendances. These findings have been supported by other studies. Therefore, supported self-management can be considered cost-effective.

Implementing supported self-management

Supported self-management can be applied to many groups, but those which have shown positive outcomes include mental health, long-term conditions with multiple comorbidities, diabetes, and weight management.

Where a commissioner has agreed with a provider to introduce or improve self-management support, the service development and improvement plan in the NHS standard contract can be a useful tool to break down the steps of development and implementation. As these self-management initiatives can vary dramatically, there is no suggested service specification wording provided in Appendix 1. However, the following is a list of things to consider as you develop the specification detail. You can specify:

- use of a patient activation measure, including:
  - o patient criteria and exception criteria;
  - o training requirements for activation measures;
  - o defined timeframes for activation measure reassessments;
  - o licencing requirements for PAM® or equivalent;
- the intervention approach, including:
  - o referral processes;
  - o delivery methods;
  - o workforce training;
  - o monitoring and evaluation methods.

Evaluation, in addition to measuring demand and uptake, considers the improvement of activation measures for people pre and post intervention. This is coupled with self-reported experiences from both those receiving support and those delivering it.

Personal health budgets

Personal health budgets are funds allocated to a person based on their individual health and care needs, identified in the personalised care and support plan process. They aim to give people more choice and control over how their health and wellbeing needs are met. These funds can be used for a variety of needs, which can be for ongoing or one-off care needs. (I examine budget types and budget setting in Chapter 7.)

Personal health budgets can be used in many ways, with some being a legal right. The legal rights for a personal health budget apply for:

- adult continuing healthcare;
- children and young people's continuing care;
- aftercare following section 117 of the Mental Health Act 1983;
- NHS wheelchairs.

Commissioners are legally obliged to provide personal health budgets for these reasons if clinically appropriate.

Other examples of use for personal health budgets that do not involve legal rights are:

- integrated budgets for health and social care packages combined (see Chapter 7);
- one-off budgets for rehabilitation or recovery aims;
- support for special educational needs and disability plans;
- specialist equipment for people with complex needs;
- transport for people requiring dialysis;
- pooled budgets for groups with a common goal, such as weight management.

Where a personal health budget offer is implemented, it sits hand in hand with the personalised care and support planning process. This planning is a prerequisite for personal health budgets. The plan sets out what it is needed for and how it will be spent. A trained professional reviews the plan with the budget holder at intervals to ensure it is still meeting their needs.

Benefits of personal health budgets

There have been many evaluations of personal health budgets, and they agree that the following general outcomes and benefits are realised (NHS England, 2024c):

- People's quality of life and wellbeing improves.
- People have more choice and control and feel more confident managing their conditions.
- People with high levels of need benefit more than those with relatively mild needs.
- The cost of care falls for people with high levels of need.
- People with personal health budgets for NHS continuing healthcare or for mental health needs spend less time in hospital than those who don't have this.
- The personalised approach tackles some avoidable health inequalities.

Implementing personal health budgets

As personal health budgets are a legal right for some people, all integrated care systems have implemented processes for these to be administrated. The challenges may come where commissioners decide to expand the offer to other health and care areas. Where examining an untested group of people for these budgets, commissioners may wish to start small, with a handful of budgets offered, then evaluate the outcomes and expand the offer to more people as confidence and evidence of success grows. The NHS England personalised care programme offers a wealth of guidance and support for those looking to improve their personal health budget offer. This includes options for training staff and navigating the regulations.

As personal health budget initiatives can vary dramatically for different care areas, there is no suggested service specification wording in Appendix 1. However, the following is a list of things to consider when developing the service specification detail:

- defining the cohort;
- determining eligibility criteria;
- mapping the service pathway, including referral processes;
- organising the budget setting process;
- having financial systems in place;
- deciding on auditing processes;
- having linked datasets where required;
- selecting evaluation measures;
- identifying workforce training requirements;

- assessing the communication and information on offer;
- making governance arrangements.

As the arrangements for personal health budgets can be quite complex, most services using them will benefit from a stand-alone service specification.

Evaluation will differ on a case-by-case basis. I would recommend that in addition to the usual demand and uptake measures, some quality measures are included that can build the case for improved health and wellbeing. These may include impact on service demand, such as demand for primary care and Accident and Emergency, or, more qualitatively, patient-reported outcome and experience measures.

Good to know: FutureNHS platform

For personalised care and many other areas of interest in healthcare, there are dedicated areas on the FutureNHS collaborative platform. This platform is a secure space for those working in the public services for health and care to connect with peers, access information, and join workspace communities.

You need to request access to most of the shared areas on FutureNHS, but these requests are usually quickly approved and access granted. Once in, you can access resources, updates, discussion forums, and more on the subject you are interested in. (See more at the FutureNHS website: https://future.nhs.uk/connect.ti.)

Commissioning for personalised care

The personalised care components should be applied with care. There are national standards and legal requirements which must be applied. And where required and possible, there should be flexibility of design and implementation approaches for improved local fit.

When examining opportunities to spread the use of personalised care, commissioners can focus on a specific group of people, such as those identified locally from the Core20PLUS5 framework

(Chapter 9) or a priority in the NHS Long Term Plan. This approach will allow commissioners and clinicians to fully map out decision making for a particular group of people, implement with confidence, evaluate, and learn from the process. The successes can then be spread and scaled up.

The expectation is that a large proportion of people receiving health and care services will potentially benefit from initiatives such as social prescribing and choice. A smaller proportion of people will be offered personalised care and support planning, supported self-management, and shared decision making. And smaller still is the proportion of people expected to be offered a personal health budget. The triangle in Figure 10.2 illustrates the estimated population proportions for each component (NHS England, 2019b). This proportion of need in some way mirrors the resources of workforce and systems required to offer each component in full. So, a personal health budget may seem a lot of work to administer, but it is used for a very small group of people so should not be a deterrent to commissioners.

Supporting structures and key enablers

To implement effective personalised care, like any transformation or improvement project, it requires that certain enablers are in place. These are worthy of consideration when seeking to improve the personalised care offer to your population. They include:

• strong system leadership – this can be a named executive on the integrated care board;

Figure 10.2: Use of personalised care

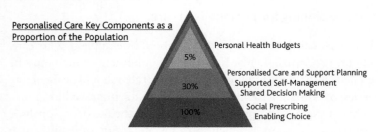

Source: NHS England (2019b) Open Government Licence v3.0

- a personalised care lead – this may be clinical or managerial. They will have a responsibility to lead change;
- clinical champions for each component – their input will ease the process;
- contracting consistency – use consistent wording, data collection methods, funding arrangements, and evaluation methods for all providers where possible. This will ease the administrative burden and be fairer for providers;
- stretched ambitions for the ICB or locality each year – for example, expand social prescribing to children and young people in year one, include personalised care and support planning requirement for all diabetes contracts in year two, and so on;
- embedded culture change – this can involve promotion and education on the benefits of personalised care and dispelling of myths about this being difficult to provide;
- co-production and workforce engagement – this is a must-do for all design and implementation of the personalised care components;
- partnership with VCSE organisations – this strengthens personalised care approaches;
- training that is consistently and frequently delivered – accredited training will be implemented where available. Training is for those delivering personalised care but also for those referring into it;
- aligned evaluation measures – this ensures the approach can produce useful learning;
- incentives to support effective personalised care delivery – for example, local CQUIN goals for personalised care and support plans.

Contracting actions for personalised care

I had the pleasure of working within the NHS England personalised care programme team for a period of time. Part of my remit was to support commissioners in planning and executing the expansion of personalised care approaches within their locality. The following are key actions that I recommended to commissioners:

- Plan a trajectory that will see 100 per cent of your contracts include at least one element of personalised care. No contract can be rationally excluded from this if they are providing care or support to people. Mapping how many contracts have personalised care components already is your starting point, and this will allow you to estimate a time period for full rollout. An ask of a provider can be quite small – for example, refer or signpost people who may benefit to social prescribing services – so you can reasonably expect this target to be met within one or two contractual years.

- Plan a trajectory for all key long-term condition pathways offering a personalised care and support plan. This may take a year or two to agree and embed if new, but many services will have a form of personalised care and support planning in place already which just needs modification to ensure it meets appropriate standards.

- Review all contracts to confirm that, where applicable, legal rights to choice are appropriately included and supported with monitoring and assurance.

- Include in strategies any opportunities for supporting growing community assets. This support enables and expands the social prescribing offer. A dedicated leader to explore and enable opportunities for community assets is recommended, and they can also be the lead for improving partnership relations.

- Choose one or two priority areas each year and focus on development in these areas. They might be supported self-management, shared decision making and/or personal health budgets.

- Establish robust reporting on personalised care approaches so you can evidence growth and evaluate impacts more effectively. Consistent data reporting is key and training providers is recommended.

Where personalised care is offered as a full suite of six components, rather than as individual stand-alone initiatives, it has full strength for realising good outcomes and being value for money.

When I was working within the NHS England palliative and end of life care programme, I shared with commissioners an example of how application of all six components may work for a single care area. Appendix 2 is an adaptation of that demonstration which illustrates how personalised care can be applied in context.

The financial impact of personalised care

Application of personalised care approaches within services can take time and resources. For example, a personalised care and support plan will take time if done well, shared decision making will make consultations slightly longer, and assessments for personal health budgets may uncover previously unidentified costs. From its earliest conception, there was some concern that personalisation of services may lead to higher costs. Of course, a conveyor belt of one size fits all will probably be quicker and slightly cheaper in the short term. But personalised care benefits show improved outcomes and value for the long term, with decreased demand on services, decreased exacerbation of conditions, improved wellbeing, and effective community-based support. More evidence is slowly emerging, and it seems to suggest that personal health budgets reduce costs or are at least cost-neutral, and the impacts on clinician's time is minimal.

Using personalised care data

The components of personalised care not only offer improved experiences and outcomes for patients, but also offer commissioners valuable information and insight into what people want and need. Personalised care and support plans show what really matters to people for their health and wellbeing goals; shared decision making and personal health budgets show what people will choose to do when faced with options; and social prescribing shows what social and emotional support needs are met in the community and where the gaps are.

Aggregating the decisions of informed individuals of a population makes it possible to commission and provide services that informed people want and need and, therefore, allocate resources more efficiently.

As personalised care becomes more business as usual, commissioners will need improved data and digital processes to cope with the collection, analysis, and sharing of information – all within interoperable, safe, and secure systems.

A personalised approach can be enhanced where people can access, view, and amend their own personal plans and preferences. There are platforms and systems for this available now, and with time the learning from the early adopters of personalised care-compatible systems will come through, and others will be able to follow this with confidence.

REFLECTIONS FOR LEADERS

Personal health budgets: Leading through uncertainty

Personal health budgets were probably the most contentious of all the personalised care components when they were first introduced. Luckily, the lack of trust in them is now starting to diminish as evidence of improved outcomes and experience is growing. One of the greatest fears was releasing money into the hands of the public – would they squander it or spend it on inappropriate things? Are PlayStations and theatre tickets real health? In reality, this type of spending was very few and far between, and the vast majority of budgets are for personal care services, such as therapy, or health aids. There is now more trust in the process with a slow growing evidence base on cost and experiences, but admittedly very little evidence on clinical outcomes.

As this is a legal right for many, and a commitment in the NHS Long Term Plan, senior leaders need to be prepared for discussions about the value and benefits of personalised care. Long term, it will be advantageous for commissioners and providers to work together on robust evaluations of their local schemes so that there is confidence about the approach.

Suggestions for success

Personalised care is a common theme, alongside health inequalities, and it is here to stay. It therefore makes sense for commissioners to begin to embed thinking about personalised care throughout their processes. That is, they should consider personalised care through every stage of the commissioning cycle. They might use personalised care data to inform the identification of need, incorporate personalised approaches into the design of services, and develop evaluation measures that examine the impact of personalised care for people and systems.

11

Commissioning for the future

Aim

This chapter discusses the impact of some of challenges that health and wellbeing commissioners and their partners face today, and those that are arising in the near future. This includes two ambitions from the NHS Long Term Plan (NHS England, 2019c), related to the ageing population and the advancement of technology. Also, the impact and learning from the COVID-19 pandemic is covered, as this has been influential in shaping health and care delivery in agile and adaptive ways and has offered a unique opportunity to accelerate change for the better. And finally, the climate change crisis is discussed, as this will have increasing impact on both demand and delivery of health and care services. Understanding these challenges helps commissioners plan for today and the future effectively.

The ageing population

What defines 'old' or 'ageing'? This is a contentious question. Generally, we refer to the older population as those aged over 65 but, as many of us will know, there can be people who are very fit at 75 years old but others at the age of 60 who are showing signs of biological older age. Instead, it is simpler to refer to the older population in terms of frailty. Frailty is the progressive loss of physical and cognitive resilience, and it is a better indicator of specialist need in older age. People who are frail are at greater risk from falls, admission to hospital, and episodes of ill health. People from some groups can be at higher risk of frailty at a younger age. This is particularly true of people in deprived areas (Stow et al, 2022). Commissioners must remain mindful of their population needs when considering 'ageing' or 'frail' populations.

Although an ageing population is seen as a problem in terms of demand, it is also a marker of success of health and social care, and the wider welfare state. In the next 25 years, the number of people aged 85 and over will double to 2.6 million (Raymond et al, 2021). We can make the obvious assumption that the ageing population will require more services to meet the growing need – and this is supported by the fact that the proportion of people aged over 75 with one or more long-term condition has risen. However, for social care, it is not quite as straightforward as that. For example, the age at which most need people need social care support has risen, with more older people living independent lives for longer. This provides some counterbalance. Here, we see that the relationship between age, health, and social care is changing. Improvements in living standards and healthcare advancements result in people staying independent and well for longer, though these same improvements mean we see a greater proportion of people with more than one complex condition as they see older age.

Planning for the older population

Using population data and forecasting assumptions, commissioners can build a picture of growing need well into the future. This analysis can aid the decision making and strategic planning for an area. Plans need to reflect trends in care needs, plus the barriers and challenges that older people face. One such barrier is age discrimination. This can take many forms, such as not receiving the same treatment offered to younger people, patronising behaviours, barriers to accessing treatment (for example, physical access for the frail or specialist support for those with dementia), personal preferences not being recognised. Therefore, as well as planning for capacity and demand, commissioners need to include improvement of culture and equality in care for older people.

The King's Fund shares key components of good provision for the older population (see Oliver et al, 2014). These are foundations of good practice and quality services that meet the needs of older people. When planning longer-term strategies for older people, commissioners should consider:

- initiatives to support:
  o healthy, active ageing and independence;
  o living well with simple or stable long-term conditions;
  o living well with complex co-morbidities, dementia, and frailty;
- implementing rapid support close to home in times of crisis;
- ensuring commissioning of:
  o good acute hospital care when needed;
  o good discharge planning and post-discharge support;
  o good rehabilitation and re-ablement after acute illness or injury;
- working with partners for high-quality nursing and residential care for those who need it;
- promoting and providing choice, control, and support towards the end of life;
- ensuring integration to provide person-centred, coordinated care.

These components embody the principles of personalised care, quality, prevention, co-ordination of care, and care closer to home.

Geriatric services

Some older people receive the same care as people of a younger age – care is matched to their need, regardless of age. An example of this is in cancer services. But some older people benefit from a more holistic approach of 'geriatric care'. Geriatric care can offer generalist care that is specialist to the unique needs of the older person. It often includes medical, psychological, and social care. In this way, it is holistic and can wrap around the needs of a patient. People's symptoms and care needs are addressed, and their care is considered as a bundle rather than addressed in silo teams. Geriatric clinicians receive training in common conditions that affect older people. This can include Parkinson's disease, Alzheimer's disease, osteoporosis, bladder problems, and polypharmacy. They are also trained and experienced in supporting frailty.

There is an argument that geriatric care is a disadvantage in that older people's needs are seen as separate from those of the wider population, and therefore are dealt with separately rather than as everyone's core business. In practice, the opposite may be true. As older age brings with it different needs, these needs can become inequalities related to ability to physically access services, social isolation, poverty, and emotional wellbeing, with the loss of loved ones. These inequalities are more readily addressed in services that identify and manage these needs directly. And as people age, they use a greater number of services. It makes sense, where possible, to integrate the response of these services under one umbrella of care and support.

Identifying people at risk

Preventative care and early support cannot be given if the people who need it are not identified until they are already very frail, have lost independence, or are presenting in crisis. Early identification of those who will benefit from targeted support is crucial. To that end, many primary care networks now work on the basis of proactive case finding. This enables the targeting of strategies to the people who will benefit most.

Frailty is a long-term condition. Severe frailty affects approximately 3 per cent of the population in England aged 65 and older, moderate frailty 12 per cent, and mild frailty 35 per cent (Clegg et al, 2016). Many studies suggest that proactive case finding, timely assessment, care planning, and targeted interventions can improve outcomes for this group.

Case finding is often a multidisciplinary approach, with many teams collaborating. To help with the process, practices can use tools which run through the risk factors stored in the coding of patient data on practice registers. This initial list is then considered in more detail by the team of professionals to identify those people at increased risk. Other methods of identifying people can include screening at clinics, such as vaccination clinics, or identification by community nurses and allied health professionals. Frailty scoring often facilitates this process, multiple frailty tools are available.

Once level of frailty is established, the cohort is stratified into risk groups. Those at highest risk are targeted first. Those in lower risk groups may receive only a simple review. This process is known as risk stratification.

When people are identified as being at a higher risk, they receive further assessments, each with a specific aim, such as:

- a falls assessment — frail people are at greater risk of falling and then have a greater risk of serious injury and slower recovery when they have fallen. People can also become socially isolated where they have a fear of falling;
- a medication review — these are to assess if there are too many prescriptions (polypharmacy), which can produce harmful effects, and to see if there are alternative medicines that are lower risk to a frail person.

Personalised care and support planning is the gold standard approach to planning effective care after assessment. Multi-agency plans that join up and consider what matters to people will be the most successful. The final step is to put into place the support and care people need to maintain independence, stay well, and reduce risk of harm. For maximum effect these are tailored interventions designed for each person according to their personal needs.

The technology revolution

Technology is beginning to play a much larger part in service delivery — it can prevent illness, enable earlier diagnosis, empower people, and ease the burden on professionals. It also has a major part to play in the way people access services, through provision of better public education, greater use of communication options with patients and service users, and the collection of relevant data to support decision making and engagement.

The NHS Long Term Plan, in Chapters 1 and 5, stresses the importance of advancement in digitally enabled care. Commissioners therefore have responsibilities for ensuring that technology solutions are considered and built into service design where it will add value. The NHS Long Term Plan commits to technological improvement efforts towards:

- digital technology for accessing advice and care;
- primary care consultations online (or by phone);
- outpatient appointments online;
- patient electronic access to health records and personalised care and support plans;
- app-based interventions;
- health monitoring technology;
- improved technology for professionals;
- digital systems to strengthen safety;
- data analysis techniques for population health assessment;
- improved information governance.

As this is a national priority, all integrated care systems must consider in their local strategic plans the long-term ambitions for improving the application of technology in their locality. The NHS Long Term Plan commitments are a good place to focus commissioning energy.

Commissioning technology for the future

There are many technologies that are tried and trusted, and there are some that are still unproven in their effectiveness and value. The job of the commissioner is to stay up to date on the technologies that have evidence while also being open to exploring new opportunities for technology as they arise. This can be a difficult balance of striving to be early adopters of groundbreaking innovation, with the risks that brings, or being the last ones to benefit.

As with any potential option for change, a business case needs to set out the need, and the proposed solution needs to demonstrate potential that is balanced with any costs and risks. Technology can be expensive, and affordability will be a challenge. The NHS and social care will struggle to keep up with rising technology costs, and therefore a value-based assessment is required to evidence an option will be worth the investment by achieving good outcomes or reducing costs elsewhere. Furthermore, the operating systems these innovations require can be technical nightmares to install into existing IT systems and processes. This can make the case for change more challenging, and it often removes some of the options for small-scale testing.

A good business case for digital solutions will include:

- the need/problem that the technology addresses;
- the predicted outcomes;
- patient safety risks;
- information governance, relating to data protection and cybersecurity;
- human factors, including human-centred design and usability;
- interoperability with other healthcare systems;
- cost-effectiveness and value for money;
- financial impact;
- how it works in a real-world setting and whether it has been tested theoretically;
- capacity to scale;
- impact on other resources, services, or workforce;
- training requirements;
- effects on the wider system and community;
- what upgrades and maintenance are required;
- regulatory requirements;
- opportunities to tackle health inequalities;
- measurability of clinical outcomes and social, economic, and behavioural benefits;
- ability to meet commercial rules and regulations.

It is the duty of commissioners and integrated care system partners to be open to technology opportunities but capitalise on them responsibly and ensure value for money.

Inequalities in the context of technology

With a thriving industry for digital healthcare solutions, it is easy to be swept away with the possibilities of technology. However, it is important to remain mindful and proactively consider the use of technology and its potential negative impact on inequalities in care. For example, where access to a service is via online booking, this creates a potential barrier for those without the means, such as a smartphone, to book an appointment. Or when considering virtual consultations, exercise classes, or follow-ups, it is necessary to consider how those who have no internet connection, compatible devices, know-how, or functioning microphones and cameras will be able to take up the offer. Also, consider people's preferences. People may not trust the technology or they may prefer face-to-face contact to make their conversations more personal and meaningful.

To mitigate against these potential limitations, commissioners can:

- consider digital access issues and address inequalities of access, skills, health literacy, trust, and privacy;
- tailor digital approaches to specific groups, such as easy-read guides or credible messages for target audiences;
- monitor the uptake and feedback from different groups as the technology is implemented;
- consider realistic behaviour changes that the technology may require, factoring in time where needed for promotion, training, and trust in new approaches.

The global pandemic

In 2020, the world was hit with the COVID-19 virus. This had massive immediate implications, but it also brought an impetus for change and a huge opportunity for learning for the future.

The impact of COVID-19 on the NHS

The NHS struggled to cope with the rising cases of people with COVID-19 in 2020. It was unprepared for the event, and it was soon apparent that there were not enough staff, beds, premises, or equipment. In addition, there was a knock-on effect for those with other health conditions, whose outpatient appointments were cancelled or routine surgeries postponed. The system leaders had to prioritise with normal services suspended. The cancellation of nearly all routine and planned care created a backlog and enormous waiting lists. These numbers soared and today we are still tackling the aftermath of people waiting for consultation and treatment.

Transformation was achieved during and following this traumatic period due to the steep learning curve we had to endure and the urgent need to adapt. The leadership at local and national level reflected this urgency with a speed and focus previously unseen. The NHS England changes in contractual regulations (including guaranteed block payments, removal of sanctions, and some national standards) also enabled providers to work in a more agile and adaptive way that wasn't previously possible. The following are just a few examples of the changes applied during the peak of the crisis and in the longer term.

At the time of the event:

- Command and control centres were quickly established to streamline decision making and information dissemination.
- Intensive care suites were established astonishingly fast in places that were not healthcare orientated.
- Mental health crisis support was upscaled and made available virtually.
- Community services and other care providers, such as hospices, stepped up to support earlier discharge.
- Appointments with clinicians were swiftly adapted to electronic virtual appointments or phone calls.
- Virus testing was rolled out to both professionals and the public.
- An immense vaccination programme was implemented. The way this was rolled out and administered by primary care was a great success. Close working with communities increased uptake.
- Communities galvanised overnight and provided support to those who were isolated – for instance, by delivering food and prescriptions to those unable to leave their homes.
- Back office and managerial staff were quickly supported to work remotely and connect with others via technology to continue their work.
- NHS England simplified NHS contracting payment terms to support rapid transformation and to allay concerns about escalating costs.

And longer-term changes include:

- acceleration of the development of virtual wards and other approaches that keep people safely at home and out of hospital;

- continued virtual appointments utilising digital technology for quick and effective communication with patients;
- strengthening and enabling of communities to support themselves effectively in times of greater need;
- improved preparedness for future pandemics in terms of learning from virus transmission and treatments;
- greater focus on identifying and addressing avoidable health inequalities;
- improved integration between health and social care to better meet population needs;
- examination of other basic needs, such as the government exploring the legal right for visitation for people in health and care settings during 2023.

The impact of COVID-19 on social care

People with social care needs suffered terribly during the pandemic. There was significant emotional distress, lack of freedom, isolation, affected access to care, deteriorating health and wellbeing, and loss of life. The social care workforce were severely affected by sickness and lack of protective equipment, and, as people were discharged more quickly from hospital, there was a significant increase in need and therefore rising demand.

On a positive note, this clear and obvious need shone a spotlight on the importance of social care, and there were many excellent models of care developed at speed to make sure vulnerable people had the support they needed. Some of the learning from the pandemic is summarised in Table 11.1 alongside some advice on how to replicate these successes.

The voluntary, community, and social enterprise sector contribution to the pandemic

At the time of the pandemic, the public services stepped up, but they were not able to meet all needs effectively. They managed to cope with the tip of the iceberg, with the voluntary, community and social enterprise (VCSE) sector and national charities providing aid to the most vulnerable in society. This included provision of food, prescriptions, comfort, and technology, among

Table 11.1: Learning for social care from the pandemic

Key learning	Replication tips
Flexible support services were able to cope best in the pandemic. They could flex teams and approaches to respond well and connect quickly and effectively with others to provide continued care.	Support teams to rip up the business-as-usual rule book when in an emergency situation. Thinking outside of the box and having flexibility to work differently is a culture change that can be encouraged in times of need.
Positive and regular communication between commissioners and providers resulted in solution-focused ways of working.	Daily sit-rep calls with key providers during times of crisis keeps everybody informed and provides opportunity for spotting issues, agreeing solutions, and peer support.
Knowing local communities and having close contact with them saved lives, as needs were identified more quickly and opportunities for wraparound care responses were co-produced.	Involve community leaders and people in the processes of managing emergency situations, and recognise the benefits they bring when they are involved and informed. Mobilise communities to support themselves.
Supported and valued unpaid carers had an assessment of their needs and were offered support to enable them to look after themselves and the person they care for.	Reach out and identify carers proactively. Provide support before ability to care is affected.
Technologies for remote monitoring kept people safe while ensuring people remained well.	Invest in telehealth and smart home technology that can support people to remain safely at home.

many other things. The VCSE sector has flexibility and a holistic approach that public sector services can struggle to match. VCSE organisations infiltrate communities and reach people who may be unable to access traditional services. They are generally trusted and respected, and they play an important role in keeping communities connected and well.

Commissioners can strengthen VCSE readiness for the next crisis by investing in their communities now. This investment can include funding, but it most certainly should include relationship strengthening, resilience building, and real involvement and collaboration.

Managing the backlog

In 2022, the government shared its commitment to the recovery of health and social care services following the pandemic – specifically the backlog of elective services. The Department of Health and Social Care worked alongside NHS England to develop a plan of action to be delivered by the new integrated care boards. Of specific note, the objectives included eliminating very long waits, speeding up diagnostics, prioritising cancer care, and improving the use of technology in outpatient care.

Chapter 7 notes that the NHS Payment Scheme for 2023–25 has been adapted to tackle waiting times in elective care and the operational planning guidance for 2023/24 includes ambitions on recovering core services and reducing waits. It is now over to those in the integrated care boards to make this a reality. However, if 2023 is anything to go by, we may see only a slow improvement in the recovery targets. The cost-of-living crisis and the staff strikes on pay have disrupted efforts to 'catch up' on waiting lists. This aim has been made even more difficult to achieve due to the effects of other industry strikes, such as railways or schools. These strikes make it difficult for staff to get to work and for patients to attend their appointments.

Although commissioners are asked to go faster with recovering core services, integrated care boards will have to factor in the other issues that can influence this and be prepared for the potential curve of greater ill health as people wait longer for diagnosis and treatment.

Environmental crisis

There is scientific consensus that, because of human behaviour, there is an environmental crisis with climate warming, melting polar ice, rising sea levels, and more frequent extreme weather events, such as flooding, drought, and heatwaves. Plus, due to our activities as humans, we are polluting our world with toxic gases in the air, chemicals in our foods, and micro-plastics in our seas.

This environmental crisis is important to health and care services because of:

- the impact it has on people's health and wellbeing;
- the impact it has **on** the circumstances of delivering health and care services;
- the environmental impact **of** delivering services.

This section examines these impacts now and for the future.

The impact on people

The potential impact of the environmental crisis on people is multiple. First, there is the physical impact on people, such as respiratory conditions due to air pollution, risk to health due to flooding or heatwave, and impacts on health due to changes in our diet, such as micro-plastics in the fish we eat. Second, as people see the crisis unfolding and are more directly impacted, it can damage emotional wellbeing and create anxiety. Poor mental health is an underestimated aspect of climate change. Third, the crisis affects our behaviours, which has knock-on effects on our health and wellbeing. We may go outdoors less or use our cars more due to extreme weather; we may eat a more limited range of foods due to risks or availability; communities may be able to offer less as resources are stretched with the pressures on social systems.

Commissioners need to be aware of these impacts. Long-term strategy planning can consider the impact of the environmental crisis on health and care future demand. System partners can plan and execute prevention of ill health strategies and improvement of self-care opportunities, and enable communities to better support people through the challenges.

The impact on care delivery

Environmental change, especially climate change, is having a growing effect on the ability of health services to operate. For example, flooding affects emergency services access to people in need, staff may struggle to get to work in adverse weather conditions, and heatwaves can affect equipment. As climate change increasingly starts to affect availability of resources, we will also see increased difficulties in obtaining supplies.

Risk assessments and planning will direct systems in the mitigation, management, and response to extreme weather events. Emergency Preparedness, Resilience and Response is the NHS approach to planning for a wide range of incidents. Extreme weather events will be a growing focus for this planning activity, and to support this the UK Health Security Agency has developed the Adverse Weather and Health Plan (UK Health Security Agency, 2023). Local plans should build on existing UK systems and measures taken by government agencies. Integrated care system plans will include integrated planning arrangements across organisations, capacity building, communication arrangements, early warning systems, and other factors important for both reducing loss of life and morbidity caused by extreme weather events and reducing the burden on healthcare services.

The environmental impact of services

Public services are contributors to the environmental problem. The delivery of services creates emissions and waste; ambulances, community nurses, and social workers drive around to get closer to people and communities, and as many as 1 in 20 cars on the road are for the NHS (Office for Health Improvement and Disparities, 2022). Hospitals and care homes are lit and heated; laundry and cleaning use large amounts of water every day; care providers use massive amounts of physical resources, and this creates wastage of paper, plastic gloves, and biowaste; and old IT hardware contributes to waste also. All these activities have a carbon footprint and/or contribute to the environmental crisis. Figure 11.1 illustrates the carbon emissions from different activities in the NHS.

Good to know: Carbon footprint

A carbon footprint is a measure of the amount of carbon dioxide released into the atmosphere because of the activities of individuals or organisations. Carbon is a greenhouse gas that is contributing to the detrimental effects of global warming. The term carbon footprint is a useful one to use

Figure 11.1: Carbon emissions in the NHS

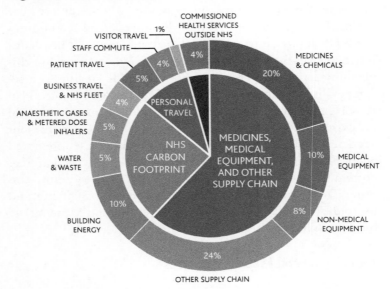

Source: Office for Health Improvement and Disparities (2022) Open Government Licence v3.0

when considering the impact of activities and the strategies to reduce environmental harm.

The concept of **net zero** means aiming to not add any carbon to the environment and to implement methods of absorbing it. The UK government has committed to reaching net zero by 2050. The public services have a role to play in reaching that target.

The NHS commitment to sustainability

The NHS Sustainability Board was established to coordinate and support environmental action. To achieve this, they have set an NHS carbon footprint target to reach net zero on *directly controllable* emissions by 2040, ten years earlier than the government commitment. The target for those emissions the NHS can only *influence* is net zero by 2045. These commitments were embedded into legislation by the Health and Care Act 2022. The *Delivering a 'Net Zero' National Health Service* report (NHS England, 2022a) is statutory guidance. It includes recommendations on practical steps for reducing emissions, such as improving estates management, electrifying transport fleets, and optimising supply chains.

Every trust and integrated care system is now required to have a green plan which sets out the aims, objectives, and plans for carbon reduction and sustainability. These are three-year strategies that support coordinated efforts to reduce emissions, in line with national trajectories, and they are signed off by the trust or system board. What is less clear is how integrated care systems will fund these initiatives. Boards will have to grapple with dwindling financial resources and may have to face difficult decisions about cutting resources or services to fund a green plan.

Action at ground level

Public services can play a large role in tackling environmental impacts. This is not always an easy route to take, but it is an essential one. It requires leadership and innovation, but it will have multiple benefits, including reducing the harm to the environment, improving people's health and wellbeing, and streamlining processes and systems, and it will contribute to a sustainable model of care.

For commissioners, there are many methods and activities for reducing environmental harms. These need to be embedded in a culture of change for maximum success. Some recommendations for different groups follow.

Professionals should:

- educate themselves and others about the risks and opportunities for reducing the carbon footprint;
- encourage commitment among colleagues to reducing their carbon footprint and reducing waste;
- talk to patients and families about how to reduce the impact of environmental harms;
- choose environmentally friendly options;
- reduce unnecessary use of consumables and energy;
- join sustainable networks.

Leaders and managers should:

- give staff permission to act on change;
- ease access to training and development for sustainability;
- collaborate with other departments to share learning and best practice;
- develop net zero ambitions at local level;
- shape team working with sustainable practices;
- embed sustainability into business cases and option appraisals.

Strategic leaders should:

- actively promote the climate action strategy that is system-wide;
- support the nominated senior leadership for the board;
- organise training and development on environmental issues;
- improve green spaces for staff;
- coordinate intelligence for preparedness in responding to extreme weather events;
- use media to communicate sustainability ambitions and to promote the approach;
- understand which local groups are particularly vulnerable to the environmental impacts;
- measure impact of green initiatives and celebrate successes;
- consider incentives in contracts and funding mechanisms to embed change related to sustainability.

Examples of sustainable initiatives

There are many good examples of sustainable initiatives across health and care systems. Here is a small sample of some those successes, and you can read more of the details on the Greener NHS web pages (NHS England, 2024b):

- use of electric vehicles in and around Greater Manchester;
- use of solar power at Milton Keynes University Hospital and Hull University Teaching Hospitals NHS Trust;
- reduction of single-use plastics at Great Ormond Street;
- the first net zero surgery at University Hospitals Birmingham;
- drone deliveries of chemotherapy to Isle of Wight patients;

- optimised use of inhalers in Worcestershire and Rochdale;
- use of cycle couriers in Oxford, Newcastle, and Sussex;
- optimised anaesthesia for surgery in Bristol;
- reduced cannulisation at Charing Cross Hospital.

REFLECTIONS FOR LEADERS

Resilience in changing times

A key attribute, or indeed skill, for senior leaders is resilience. Given the changing pressures for public services, this is more important than ever. Resilience is the ability to recover from, adapt to, and grow from difficulties. When facing adversity, resilient leaders can find opportunities for positive change while supporting others around them to manage and emerge from challenges.

Four ways to build and strengthen your resilience are:

- Reflect and assess – this means understanding yourself and your strengths as a leader. Knowing what you are good at and what support you need in other areas will only make you a stronger leader.

- Identify learning and growth opportunities – resilience is like a muscle that when used gets stronger. Learning and growing from challenging situations helps us navigate the next ones.

- Be purpose driven – keep the end vision in mind and continuously reassess your course to make sure it is still on track to meet that aim.

- Cultivate relationships – no person is an island, and we need the strength, guidance, and different perspectives of others to meet and greet the challenges we face. Grow your network to become a stronger and more capable leader.

Resilience is not about being tough, but about being comfortable with being uncomfortable in times of uncertainty.

Suggestions for success

What this chapter has shown is that although we can plan, design, deliver, and evaluate for improvement, we always need to build in flexibility for long-range projections and the unexpected. Whether that is the slow but foreseen ageing population and technological advances, or the unpredictable climate events and global pandemics, commissioners need to be ready to adapt and learn. Viewing the process as a cycle will help with that approach – that is, no process of commissioning ends but instead it evolves to improve or to meet new need and changing times.

A model of outcomes-based commissioning

Summarising an effective approach

We have come on a long journey through the stages of commissioning and the key ingredients that make any commissioning practice a greater success regarding good outcomes and experiences for people and their communities. In this concluding chapter, I bring together the priority aspects in a model for good commissioning. Although all the individual model components require in-depth understanding and practical knowledge, I would suggest the model can act as a simple memory aid when considering new commissioning projects or programmes – commissioners can ask: have all the aspects of the model been considered adequately and employed appropriately?

This model is more effectively applied to larger commissioning projects. A proportional approach will be needed for smaller commissioning projects.

The aim is to strive towards outcomes-based commissioning. I suggest that today, compared with ten years ago, what constitutes good commissioning has significantly changed. It is now a difficult balance between achieving quality outcomes for people and achieving sustainability in a resource-challenged environment. This means embracing change and innovation to tailor solutions for improving local outcomes. What this will look like will be quite different from area to area, but the focus for commissioners is to achieve good or improved outcomes for the population through defining, planning, and contracting health and care services.

The model

The model (shown in Figure 12.1) includes three **output pillars**. These pillars are essential – each one must be in place to support the aim of outcomes-based commissioning. The foundation for these pillars is provided by **enabling bricks**. You could remove a few of the enabling bricks, but the model would be less 'stable' and potentially less likely to succeed or to stand the test of time.

Figure 12.1: Model of outcomes-based commissioning

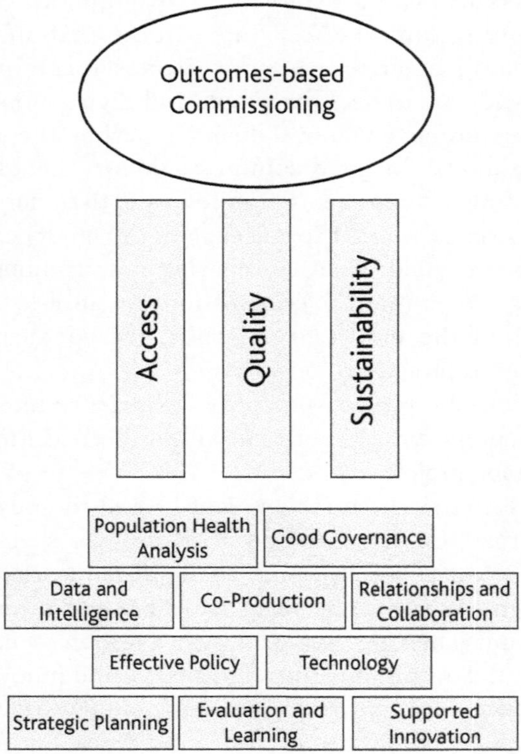

The output pillars

The output pillars of outcomes-based commissioning are **Access**, **Quality**, and **Sustainability**.

Access

The Access output pillar ensures that services, care, and support are accessible to those who need it. Here, commissioners are looking to ensure that services are provided at the right time, in the right place, and for the right people. Access as an output seeks to reduce avoidable health and care inequalities.

Quality

The Quality output pillar relates to the vital requirement of ensuring services, care, and support are effective, safe, holistic, and personalised to meet people's individual needs. The quality output pillar is aligned with achieving the desired outcomes and takes account of people's needs as a whole.

Sustainability

The Sustainability output pillar is vital for ensuring services, care, and support are future-fit and supported for continued delivery, now and in the future. This pillar considers funding, but equally it considers the sustainability of aspects such as workforce, technology requirements, capacity and demand, and the environmental impact.

The enabling bricks

The output pillars need strong supporting structures to ensure they are implemented and achieved effectively – these are the enabling bricks. The bricks are not all essential, but without the majority in place the pillars will lose stability and service design is less likely to be optimal. Like any brick tower, if you start pulling a few out, the tower may topple. Commissioners should seek to implement as many bricks as possible to create a firm enabling structure. The enabling bricks are:

- population health analysis – processes to identify and understand local needs;
- good governance – processes which safeguard success, such as through effective boards and contracts;
- data and intelligence – support for understanding need, effective design, and meaningful evaluation;
- co-production – proactive involvement of people and communities in developing effective change;
- relationships and collaboration – supported joint working for achieving shared goals and system improvements;
- effective policy – use of local and national policy that provides clarity on good practice;
- technology – harnessing of the technological opportunities for enhancing service design and delivery;
- strategic planning – future-forward planning that incorporates system-wide goals and acknowledges future challenges;
- evaluation and learning – information sharing and transparency, contributing to sharing the responsibility for continuous improvement;
- supported innovation – openness to new approaches in times of change.

Although, as I have acknowledged throughout, commissioning can be challenging at times, I believe that with the application of this commissioning model, any health and care service can be designed to achieve the three output pillars and deliver better health and wellbeing outcomes for the population.

APPENDIX 1

Personalised care in service specifications

The following wording has been adapted from the *Finance, Commissioning and Contracting Handbook for Personalised Care* (NHS England, 2019b), which I authored on behalf of NHS England in 2019.

Personalised care service requirements often need to sit within service specifications for a care pathway or service. They are a single part of a wider whole. It is important to ensure that the requirements for personalised care are captured effectively. Commissioners may find the example wording in the boxes helpful when considering shared decision making, personalised care and support planning, and social prescribing.

This example wording will require modifying to meet local requirements, but offer a useful start as specifications are developed or revised.

Box A2.1: Example service specification wording for shared decision making

Shared decision making is a process in which individuals and clinicians work together to understand and decide what tests, treatments, or support packages are most suitable bearing in mind a person's own circumstances. It brings together the individual's expertise about themselves and what is important to them together with the clinician's knowledge about the benefits and risks of the options. This means that lay expertise is given the same value as clinical expertise.

To be successful, it relies on two sources of expertise:

- the [INSERT health professional] as an expert on the effectiveness, probable benefits, and potential harms of treatment options for [INSERT pathway]; and
- the individual as an expert on themselves, their social circumstances, attitudes to illness and risk, values and preferences, and the supplied knowledge of the latest evidence.

Shared decision making enables individuals to align their preferences to treatment options that are clinically valid. It does not mean that people can choose clinical treatments that have no evidence base. For this service, the key options are as follows:

- [INSERT option];
- [INSERT option];
- [INSERT option].

The Provider must:

- implement shared decision making for [INSERT eligible patients];
- have a clear written protocol in place for shared decision making and its use in the [INSERT care pathway];
- ensure applicable staff are trained in the skills of shared decision making, and this entails [INSERT requirements, such as type of training and frequency].

The Provider will ensure that the patients are prepared by [INSERT how people are prepared and supported].

The Provider will identify a named clinical champion, and they will be given appropriate time to support the implementation of the new approach for interacting with service users.

Box A2.2: Example service specification wording for personalised care and support planning

Personalised care and support planning encourages care professionals and people with long-term conditions and their carers to work together to clarify and understand what is important to that individual. They agree goals, identify support needs, develop and implement action plans, and monitor progress. This is a planned and continuous process, not a one-off event.

Personalised care and support planning is a process in which the person with a long-term condition is an active and equal partner. The process should normally be recorded in a written plan. This process recognises the person's skills and strengths, as well as their experiences and the things that matter the most to them. It addresses issues and identifies outcomes and actions to resolve these.

The Provider must:

1. Offer personalised care and support planning to people 'INSERT criteria].
2. Where an offer of personalised care and support planning is accepted, ensure the five criteria are applied, including:
   - People are central in developing and agreeing their personalised care and support plan.
   - People have proactive, personalised conversations which focus on what matters to them, paying attention to their needs and wider health and wellbeing.
   - People agree the health and wellbeing outcomes they want to achieve.
   - Each person has a sharable, personalised care and support plan which records what matters to them, their outcomes, and how they will be achieved.
   - People are able to formally and informally review their personalised care and support plan.

The Provider will ensure applicable staff are trained in the skills of personalised care and support planning and this entails [INSERT requirements, such as type of training and frequency] OR the Provider will identify a personalised care and support planning coordinator who has received appropriate training.

The Provider will ensure that the patients are prepared for their personalised care and support planning process by [INSERT how people are prepared and supported].

The Provider will identify a named clinical champion, and they will be given appropriate time to support the implementation of the new way of interacting with service users.

Where an offer of a personalised care and support planning is declined, the Provider will record the reason for the refusal and make this information available to the commissioner for analysis.

Box A2.3: Example service specification wording for social prescribing

Social prescribing is a way for local agencies to refer people to a link worker. As members of the primary care network team of health professionals, link workers give people time, focusing on 'what matters to me', and take a holistic and culturally appropriate approach to address people's health and wellbeing. They provide personalised support to individuals, their families, and carers to take control of their health and wellbeing, live independently, improve their health access and outcomes, and connect to community groups and statutory services for practical and emotional support.

The Provider must:

1. Implement a process for identifying people with [INSERT criteria] need
2. Offer a social prescribing referral to all people identified with potential need in 1 within [X] working days

The Provider will identify people for social prescribing following assessment of needs and will ensure the individual is aware of the referral and the benefits it may have. The Provider will liaise with social prescribing services to ensure they have appropriate access to link workers for the service cohorts needs – for example, accessibility.

Where an offer of referral is declined, the Provider will record the reason for the refusal of referral and make this information available to the commissioner and the social prescribing service for analysis.

APPENDIX 2

Personalised care in context: A hypothetical example

The following information aims to demonstrate, using a fictional case study, how the comprehensive model for personalised care can be applied within a service. This example demonstrates the potential impact in the palliative and end of life care context.

The scenario

Mrs C. is a widow who lives on her own. She has three children and the nearest lives two hours' drive away. She has long-standing COPD, but over the past year this has become increasingly severe, and she has needed two hospital admissions. Two months ago, she was diagnosed with lung cancer with secondaries to her bone and liver. The following illustrates the opportunities and benefits of personalised care as seen through Mrs C.'s eyes.

To support effective personalised care, in an ideal scenario, Mrs C. would be involved in the coordination of her care and options. Assessment and subsequent planning would be effectively shared so that Mrs C. does not have to repeatedly tell her story and her care would join up to ensure a comprehensive and integrated response. This coordination can be led by any appropriate professional and may be the responsibility of a multidisciplinary team.

Shared decision making

There are many opportunities and critical points for shared decision making for Mrs C., which include:

- deciding whether to accept palliative treatment for her lung cancer;
- deciding what level of treatment/intervention she would wish in the event of another exacerbation of COPD – including hospital admission – discussion about the thresholds for these decisions – for example, severity of breathlessness and availability of carers;
- deciding whether to record her wishes about future care at this stage, including decisions about cardiopulmonary resuscitation;
- deciding what sorts of intervention she would prefer for symptom management, knowing their side effects.

Personalised care and support planning

The personalised care and support planning process for Mrs C. can include:

- holistic assessment of physical, psychological, emotional, social, and spiritual needs;
- discussion about what matters most to her;
- discussion about how this will be incorporated into a personalised care and support plan, and discussion about when and how a review is triggered;
- discussions about the level of personal care she needs now – for example, she decides that she only needs morning carers;
- summarising the decisions arising from these discussions into a format that can be shared with professionals, Mrs C., and those who matter to her, to be used to guide delivery of care, treatment, and support;
- planning for her personal welfare – such as making a will and discussing funeral arrangements with her children;
- ensuring that key information about her plan is shared with those who might need it, including her GP and community nurse, hospital staff, ambulance services, NHS111, GP out of hours services, her family and/or whoever is close to her locally, and any specialist services involved, such as respiratory, oncology, and palliative care.

Advance care planning is a form of personalised care and support planning. It is a voluntary process of person-centred discussion between an individual and their care providers about their preferences and priorities for future care, while they have the mental capacity for meaningful conversation about these. Mrs C. can be more confident that what matters most to her will be known and considered as part of treatment decisions in the event of an emergency situation or if she becomes unable to fully participate in decision making. She is particularly keen to have these conversations, because her husband had not done so, and she had found it difficult at times to have to contribute to decisions on his behalf by guessing, rather than knowing, his wishes.

Enabling choice

The benefits of choice for Mrs C. include:

- Awareness of choices available to her in terms of choice of provider and services. Where referred for the first time, Mrs C. can use the e-Referral system supported by primary care staff. Using this system, Mrs C. can exercise her right to choose a hospital or consultant team.
- If Mrs C. is not be satisfied with the quality of personal carers that she has coming to her each morning, the use of personal health budgets could enable her to exercise greater choice and control over this aspect of her life.

Social prescribing and community-based support

In support of routine care, Mrs C. can be referred to social prescribing by her GP and a link worker can offer holistic support, including signposting to:

- a weekly local health walk, giving Mrs C. the opportunity to connect socially while exercising safely;
- a volunteer who helps with her shopping once a week;
- a community centre for a weekly lunch club, giving Mrs C. the opportunity to connect with the community and avoid social isolation;
- lessons on how to use an iPad so that she can skype her family regularly. This has multidimensional benefits: not only is Mrs

C. able to speak with her family, including her grandchildren more easily, but her family feel more reassured of her wellbeing via video, as they can see her. She can also take advantage of remote consultations with her GP and specialist teams.

Supported self-management

Supported self-management to support Mrs C. is in the form of:

- health coaching sessions based at her GP surgery. Here, she starts working on symptom management techniques for breathlessness, pain, and anxiety.

As a result of this supported self-management, Mrs C. feels more confident about joining the activities offered through social prescribing, and this has resulted in an increase in her self-confidence and willingness to get out and about, and to socialise with others.

Personal health budgets

Personal health budgets are not a legal right for palliative and end of life care, but the local integrated care system has widened the offer because they see a significant benefit for people. For Mrs C. this means:

- She is offered a personal health budget as direct payment. She uses this to replace the daily carer with an arrangement to pay her neighbour to check in with her every day and be on standby in case she's needed. Mrs C. prefers this because she doesn't need a carer to wash and dress her, she just needs someone to come in and check on her at home every day. She feels more confident knowing it is her neighbour. This results in a much lower cost to the commissioner.
- As Mrs C.'s disease progresses, she becomes more dependent on others to help her. Her personal health budget is increased following a review of her personalised care and support plan, recognising her need for additional support. This enables Mrs C. to pay another neighbour to pop in to check on her in the evenings as well. This provides Mrs C. with greater security and keeps her living well and independently at home.

APPENDIX 3

NHS Constitution

The NHS Constitution principles

The NHS Constitution (Department of Health and Social Care, 2021) outlines the rights of patients and the pledges made by the NHS for England. All NHS bodies, including privately owned organisations providing for the NHS, must abide by the constitution rules by law. Within this constitution, the NHS is founded on a common set of principles and values. These apply to the people it serves and the staff working within it.

There are seven guiding principles:

1. The NHS provides a comprehensive service, available to all – a comprehensive service includes a commitment to improve, prevent, diagnose, and treat physical and mental health problems, and this is available to all people.
2. Access to NHS services is based on clinical need, not an individual's ability to pay – NHS services are free of charge except in limited circumstances.
3. The NHS aspires to the highest standards of excellence and professionalism – services will be high quality, safe, and effective. Staff will be valued, skilled, and developed. Respect and dignity will be at the core of how staff and patients are treated.
4. The patient will be at the heart of everything the NHS does – patients will be supported to manage their own health, have their personal preferences met, will be involved in, and consulted on decisions about their care, and their feedback will be sought.

5. The NHS works across organisational boundaries – the NHS will work with other organisations in the interests of patients and local communities. This includes the local authority, private, and voluntary sector organisations.
6. The NHS is committed to providing best value for taxpayer's money – resources will be used in a way that is fair, effective, and sustainable, in a way that benefits people.
7. The NHS is accountable to the public, communities, and patients that it serves – the government sets the framework for the NHS, but it is the local NHS, patients, and clinicians who make most of the decisions about care. With a system of responsibility, the NHS will be transparent and clear to the public, patients, and staff about the decisions it makes.

In addition to these principles, you can read more about the NHS values, and the pledges to patients and NHS staff (see Department of Health and Social Care, 2021). Pledges are not legal rights.

Patient legal rights

The NHS Constitution sets out legal patient rights and information on what to do if these legal rights are not met. A summary of these rights include:

- access to health services;
- quality of care and environment;
- nationally approved treatments, drugs, and programmes;
- respect, consent, and confidentiality;
- informed choice;
- involvement in your healthcare and the NHS;
- complaint and redress.

The full details of each are found in the NHS Constitution publication. You will notice that these reflect the principles of the constitution. You can also read more about the legal rights for NHS staff which include safe and good working environments, fair pay, and equal treatment (see Department of Health and Social Care, 2021).

Responsibilities of the patients and public, and of staff

Because the NHS belongs to us all, we as patients have a responsibility to it, and to maximising the benefits for ourselves. These responsibilities are as follows:

- Recognise that you can make a significant contribution to your own, and your family's, good health and wellbeing, and take personal responsibility for it.
- Register with a general practice, as this is the main point of access to NHS care.
- Treat NHS staff and other patients with respect and recognise that violence, or the causing of nuisance or disturbance on NHS premises, could result in prosecution.
- Provide accurate information about your health, condition, and status.
- Keep appointments or cancel within reasonable time.
- Follow the course of treatment which you have agreed, and talk to your clinician if you find this difficult.
- Participate in important public health programmes, such as vaccination.
- Ensure that those closest to you are aware of your wishes about organ donation.
- Give feedback – both positive and negative – about your experiences and the treatment and care you have received.

The constitution also includes the responsibilities of staff, including legal duties such as professional accountability, duty of care, and duty to not discriminate against patients or staff.

References

Anandaciva, S. (2023) *How does the NHS compare to the health care systems of other countries?* The King's Fund [Online] Available from: www.kingsfund.org.uk/publications/nhs-compare-health-care-systems-other-countries [Accessed August 2023].

Asaria, M., Doran, T. and Cookson, R.J. (2016) 'The costs of inequality: whole-population modelling study of lifetime inpatient hospital costs in the English National Health Service by level of neighbourhood deprivation', *Epidemiology Community Health*, 70(10): 990–996.

Azamar-Alonso, A., Costa, A.P., Huebner, L.A. and Tarride, J.E. (2019) 'Electronic referral systems in health care: a scoping review', *Clinicoeconomics Outcomes Research*, 11: 325–333.

Barker, I., Steventon, A. and Deeny, S. (2017) 'Patient activation is associated with fewer visits to both general practice and emergency departments: a cross-sectional study of patients with long-term conditions', *Clinical Medicine*, 17(s3): s15. doi: 10.7861/clinmedicine.17-3s-s15

BBC (2020) 'Not racist v anti-racist: what's the difference?' [Online] Available from: www.bbc.co.uk/bitesize/articles/zs9n2v4 [Accessed August 2023].

Bell, T. (2021) 'Here's a simple way', tweet, 17 November [Online] Available from: https://twitter.com/TorstenBell/status/1461039871510958085 [Accessed April 2024].

Bevan, G., Karanikolos, M., Exley, J., Connolly, S. and Mays, N. (2014) *The four health systems of the UK: how do they compare?* Nuffield Trust and Health Foundation [Online] Available from: www.nuffieldtrust.org.uk/research/the-four-health-systems-of-the-uk-how-do-they-compare [Accessed August 2023].

Cabinet Office (2016) 'The Commissioning Academy' [Online] Available from: www.gov.uk/guidance/the-commissioning-academy-information#what-is-commissioning [Accessed August 2023].

Clegg, A., Bates, C., Young, J., Ryan, R., Nichols, L., Teale, E.A., Mohammed, M., Parry, J. and Marshall, T. (2016) 'Development and validation of an electronic frailty index using routine primary care electronic health record data', *Age and Ageing*, 45(3): 353–360.

Coalition for Personalised Care (2023) 'Co-production' [Online] Available from: www.coalitionforpersonalisedcare.org.uk/co-production/ [Accessed August 2023].

CQC (Care Quality Commission) (2022) 'The five questions we ask' [Online] Available from: www.cqc.org.uk/about-us/how-we-do-our-job/five-key-questions-we-ask [Accessed August 2023].

Curry, N., Castle-Clarke, S. and Hemmings, N. (2018) *What can England learn from the long-term care system in Japan?* Nuffield Trust [Online] Available from: www.nuffieldtrust.org.uk/sites/default/files/2018-05/1525785625_learning-from-japan-final.pdf [Accessed August 2023].

Department for Levelling Up, Housing and Communities and Department for Education (2022) *Early Help System Guide* [Online] Available from: https://assets.publishing.service.gov.uk/government/uploads/system/uploads/attachment_data/file/1078299/Early_Help_System_Guide.pdf [Accessed August 2023].

Department of Health (2010) *Measuring social value: how five social enterprises did it* [Online] Available from: https://assets.publishing.service.gov.uk/government/uploads/system/uploads/attachment_data/file/215895/dh_122354.pdf [Accessed August 2023].

Department of Health and Social Care (2021) 'NHS Constitution for England' [Online] Available from: www.gov.uk/government/publications/the-nhs-constitution-for-england [Accessed August 2023].

Department of Health and Social Care (2022a) 'Adult social care charging reform: further details' [Online] Available from: www.gov.uk/government/publications/build-back-better-our-plan-for-health-and-social-care/adult-social-care-charging-reform-further-details [Accessed June 2023].

Department of Health and Social Care (2022b) *Women's health strategy for England* [Online] Available from: www.gov.uk/gov ernment/publications/womens-health-strategy-for-england [Accessed August 2023].

Department of Health and Social Care (2023) 'NHS Choice Framework – what choices are available to you in your NHS care' [Online] Available from: www.gov.uk/government/publi cations/the-nhs-choice-framework [Accessed August 2023].

Diabetes UK (2021) 'Ethnicity and type 2 diabetes' [Online] Available from: www.diabetes.org.uk/diabetes-the-basics/types-of-diabetes/type-2/diabetes-ethnicity [Accessed August 2023].

Durand, M.A., Carpenter, L., Dolan, H., Bravo, P., Mann, M., Bunn, F. and Elwyn, G. (2014) 'Do interventions designed to support shared decision-making reduce health inequalities? A systematic review and meta-analysis', *PLOS ONE*, 9(4): 94670. doi: 10.1371/journal.pone.0094670

Elwyn, G. (2024) 'collaboRATE' [Online] Available from: www. glynelwyn.com/collaborate.html [Accessed January 2024].

Fenney, D., Thorstensen-Woll, C. and Bottery, S. (2023) *Caring in a complex world*, The King's Fund [Online] Available from: www. kingsfund.org.uk/publications/unpaid-carers-caring-complex-world [Accessed August 2023].

Finch, D. (2022) 'The cost-of-living crisis is a health emergency too', *The Health Foundation* [Online] Available from: www.hea lth.org.uk/news-and-comment/blogs/the-cost-of-living-crisis-is-a-health-emergency-too [Accessed August 2023].

Fuller, C. (2022) *Next steps for integrating primary care: the Fuller Stocktake Report*, NHS England and NHS Improvement [Online] Available from: www.england.nhs.uk/wp-content/uploads/2022/05/next-steps-for-integrating-primary-care-fuller-stockt ake-report.pdf [Accessed August 2023].

Fytche, I. (2023) 'District councils are the NHS's natural health improvement partners', *Health Service Journal*, 4 July [Online] Available from: www.hsj.co.uk/integrated-care/district-counc ils-are-the-nhss-natural-health-improvement-partners/7035090. article [Accessed August 2023].

Gomez, L.E. and Bernet, P. (2019) 'Diversity improves performance and outcomes', *Journal of the National Medical Association*, 111(4): 383–392.

Healthcare Financial Management Association (2021) *Benefits realisation:* how does a benefits realisation approach support the delivery of value? HFMA briefing [Online] Available from: www.hfma.org.uk/docs/default-source/publications/briefings/attach-6-encl-1-benefits-realisation-final.pdf?sfvrsn=f5ba73e7_0 [Accessed August 2023].

Healthcare Financial Management Association (2023) *Health inequalities: establishing the case for change*, HFMA briefing [Online] Available from: www.hfma.org.uk/docs/default-source/publi cations/briefings/hfma-health-inequalities-establishing-the-case-for-change-may-2023.pdf?sfvrsn=e56a4de7_0 [Accessed July 2023].

Healthwatch (2020) 'How to co-produce with seldom-heard groups' [Online] Available from: https://network.healthwatch.co.uk/guidance/2020-10-26/how-to-co-produce-seldom-heard-groups [Accessed December 2023].

Hewitt, N. (2018) 'Social exclusion kills: society's healthcare systems can and must help', *College of Medicine and Integrated Health* [Online] Available from: https://collegeofmedicine.org.uk/social-exclusion-kills-societys-healthcare-systems-can-and-must-help/ [Accessed August 2023].

Hewitt, P. (2023) *The Hewitt Review: an independent review of integrated care systems*, Department of Health and Social Care [Online] Available from: www.gov.uk/government/publicati ons/the-hewitt-review-an-independent-review-of-integrated-care-systems [Accessed August 2023].

Infrastructure and Projects Authority (2017) *Guide for effective benefits management in major projects* [Online] Available from: www.gov.uk/government/publications/guide-for-effective-benefits-management-in-major-projects [Accessed August 2023].

Jayatilleke, N. (2020) 'Health equity audit guidance published for NHS screening providers and commissioners' [Online] Available from: https://phescreening.blog.gov.uk/2020/08/21/health-equity-audit-guidance-published-for-nhs-screening-provid ers-and-commissioners/ [Accessed August 2023].

Kilvert, A. (2023) 'Health inequalities and diabetes', *Practical Diabetes*, 40(1): 19–24a.

Kotter, J.P. (1996) *Leading change*, Harvard Business School Press.

Local Government Association (2017) *Bright Futures: getting the best for children, young people and families* [Online] Available from: www.local.gov.uk/sites/default/files/documents/ Bright%20Futures%20-%20LGA%20children%27s%20soc ial%20care%207%20point%20plan__15_8_2017.pdf [Accessed August 2023].

Macpherson, W. (1999) 'Sir William Macpherson's definition of institutional racism', *Health Service Journal*, 4 March [Online] Available from: www.hsj.co.uk/home/sir-william-macphers ons-definition-of-institutional-racism/29259.article [Accessed August 2023].

Maslow, A.H. (1943) 'A theory of human motivation', *Psychological Review*, 50(4): 370–396.

Moberly, T. (2018) 'Scrap NHS competition rules, BMA says', *BMJ News* [Online] Available from: www.bmj.com/content/ 361/bmj.k2791 [Accessed January 2024].

National Audit Office (2011) 'Decommissioning toolkit: principles for successful decommissioning' [Online] Available from: www. nao.org.uk/decommissioning/before-you-start/principles-for-successful-decommissioning/ [Accessed August 2023].

National Audit Office (nd) 'Decommissioning toolkit contents' [Online] Available from: www.nao.org.uk/decommissioning-toolkit-contents/ [Accessed April 2024].

Nex, K. (2023) 'Social investment funding: a lifeline for the NHS', *Health Service Journal*, 20 June [Online] Available from: www.hsj. co.uk/finance-and-efficiency/social-investment-funding-a-lifel ine-for-the-nhs/7035026.article [Accessed August 2023].

NHS Confederation (2022) 'NHS leaders facing real-terms cut in funding', Press release [Online] Available from: www.nhscon fed.org/news/nhs-leaders-facing-real-terms-cut-funding-and-impossible-choices-over-which-areas-patient-care [Accessed January 2024].

NHS Confederation (2024) 'Integrated Care Systems Network', [Online] Available from: www.nhsconfed.org/ics [Accessed January 2024].

NHS Digital (2023a) 'Community services statistics' [Online] Available from: https://digital.nhs.uk/data-and-information/ publications/statistical/community-services-statistics-for-child ren-young-people-and-adults [Accessed August 2023].

NHS Digital (2023b) 'Mental health services monthly statistics' [Online] Available from: https://digital.nhs.uk/data-and-info rmation/data-tools-and-services/data-services/mental-hea lth-data-hub/dashboards/mental-health-services-mont hly-statistics#mental-health-time-series-data-dashboard [Accessed August 2023].

NHS Digital (2023c) 'Service on a page SUS+' [Online] Available from: https://digital.nhs.uk/services/secondary-uses-service-sus/service-on-a-page [Accessed August 2023].

NHS England (2016) *Securing meaningful choice for patients: CCG planning and improvement guide* [Online] Available from: PPB-13-choice-planning-guidance.pdf (rossendalecommunitydirectory.co.uk) [Accessed August 2023].

NHS England (2019a) *A five-year framework for GP contract reform to implement the NHS long term plan* [Online] Available from: www.england.nhs.uk/publication/gp-contract-five-year-framework/ [Accessed January 2024].

NHS England (2019b) *Finance, commissioning and contracting handbook for personalised care* [Online] Available from: www.engl and.nhs.uk/wp-content/uploads/2019/08/finance-commission ing-contracting-handbook-personalised-care-v2.1.pdf [Accessed February 2024].

NHS England (2019c) *The NHS long term plan* [Online] Available from: www.longtermplan.nhs.uk/ [Accessed August 2023].

NHS England (2019d) *Universal personalised care: implementing the comprehensive model* [Online] Available from: www.england.nhs.uk/wp-content/uploads/2019/01/universal-personalised-care.pdf [Accessed August 2023].

NHS England (2021a) *Building strong integrated care systems everywhere: ICS implementation guidance on partnerships with the voluntary, community and social enterprise sector* [Online] Available from: www.england.nhs.uk/wp-content/uploads/2021/06/B0905-vcse-and-ics-partnerships.pdf [Accessed August 2023].

NHS England (2021b) *Community services currency guidance: frailty and last year of life* [Online] Available from: www.england.nhs.uk/wp-content/uploads/2021/03/21-22NT_Community-Frai lty-and-Last-Year-of-Life.pdf [Accessed August 2023].

NHS England (2022a) *Delivering a 'Net Zero' National Health Service* [Online] Available from: www.england.nhs.uk/greener nhs/wp-content/uploads/sites/51/2022/07/B1728-delivering-a-net-zero-nhs-july-2022.pdf [Accessed August 2023].

NHS England (2022b) *Tackling inequalities in healthcare access, experience and outcomes* [Online] Available from: www.england. nhs.uk/wp-content/uploads/2022/07/B1779-Actionable-Insig hts-Tackling-inequalities-in-healthcare-access-experience-and-outcomes-guidance-July-202.pdf [Accessed July 2023].

NHS England (2023a) *Integrated care boards in England* [Online] Available from: www.england.nhs.uk/publication/integrated-care-boards-in-england/#map [Accessed June 2023].

NHS England (2023b) 'Introduction to the NHS Payment Scheme webinar', April 2023 [Online] Available from: www. england.nhs.uk/pay-syst/nhs-payment-scheme/ [Accessed August 2023].

NHS England (2023c) 'NHS data model and dictionary: Community Services Data Set' [Online] Available from: www.datadictionary. nhs.uk/index.html [Accessed January 2024].

NHS England (2023d) 'NHS equality, diversity, and inclusion improvement plan' [Online] Available from: www.england.nhs. uk/long-read/nhs-equality-diversity-and-inclusion-improvem ent-plan/ [Accessed February 2024].

NHS England (2023e) *NHS long term workforce plan* [Online] Available from: www.england.nhs.uk/publication/nhs-long-term-workforce-plan/ [Accessed August 2023].

NHS England (2023f) *2023/25 NHS Payment Scheme* [Online] Available from: www.england.nhs.uk/wp-content/uplo ads/2023/03/23-25-NHS-Payment-Scheme.pdf [Accessed August 2023].

NHS England (2024a) 'Core20PLUS5 (adults) – an approach to reducing healthcare inequalities' [Online] Available from: www. england.nhs.uk/about/equality/equality-hub/national-hea lthcare-inequalities-improvement-programme/core20plus5/ [Accessed January 2024].

NHS England (2024b) 'Greener NHS: system progress' [Online] Available from: www.england.nhs.uk/greenernhs/whats-alre ady-happening/ [Accessed January 2024].

NHS England (2024c) 'Personalised care: evidence and case studies' [Online] Available from: www.england.nhs.uk/personali sedcare/evidence-and-case-studies/ [Accessed January 2024].

NHS England (2024d) 'Personalised care' [Online] Available from: www.england.nhs.uk/personalisedcare/ [Accessed January 2024].

NHS England (2024e) 'Shared care records' [Online] Available from: www.england.nhs.uk/digitaltechnology/connecteddigital systems/shared-care-records/ [Accessed January 2024].

NHS England (2024f) 'The equality and health inequalities hub: case studies' [Online] Available from: www.england. nhs.uk/about/equality/equality-hub/case-studies/ [Accessed January 2024].

NHS England (2024g) 'What is commissioning?' [Online] Available from: www.england.nhs.uk/commissioning/what-is-commissioning/ [Accessed January 2024].

NHS England and NHS Improvement (2020) *Mental health currency review* [Online] Available from: www.england.nhs.uk/ wp-content/uploads/2021/02/21-22_Mental_health_currency _review.pdf [Accessed August 2023].

NHS England and NHS Improvement (2021) *Integrated care systems: design framework* [Online] Available from: www.engl and.nhs.uk/wp-content/uploads/2021/06/B0642-ics-design-framework-june-2021.pdf [Accessed January 2024].

NHS England and NHS Improvement (2022a) *Introduction to the 2022/23 national tariff* [Online] Available from: www.england. nhs.uk/wp-content/uploads/2022/04/Introduction-to-the-2022-23-tariff.pdf [Accessed August 2023].

NHS England and NHS Improvement (2022b) *Roadmap for integrating specialised services within integrated care systems* [Online] Available from: www.england.nhs.uk/wp-content/uploads/ 2022/05/PAR1440-specialised-commissioning-roadmap-adden dum-may-2022.pdf [Accessed June 2023].

Office for Health Improvement and Disparities (2022) 'Climate and health: applying All Our Health' [Online] Available from: www.gov.uk/government/publications/climate-change-applying-all-our-health/climate-and-health-applying-all-our-health [Accessed August 2023].

Oliver, D., Foot, C. and Humphries, R. (2014) *Making our health and care systems fit for an ageing population*, The King's Fund [Online] Available from: www.kingsfund.org.uk/publications/making-our-health-and-care-systems-fit-ageing-population [Accessed August 2023].

Patient ALS Partner (2024) 'SDM-Q-9 / SDM-Q-Doc' [Online] Available from: www.patient-als-partner.de/index.php?article_id=20&clang=2/ [Accessed January 2024].

Polley, M. and Pilkington, K. (2017) *A review of the evidence assessing impact of social prescribing on healthcare demand and cost implications*, Technical report, University of Westminster [Online] Available from: westminsterresearch.westminster.ac.uk/item/q1455/a-review-of-the-evidence-assessingimpact-of-social-prescribing-on-healthcare-demand-and-cost-implications [Accessed August 2023].

Public Health England (2019) *PHE strategy 2020 to 2025* [Online] Available from: www.gov.uk/government/publications/phe-strategy-2020-to-2025 [Accessed February 2024].

Raymond, A., Bazeer, N., Barclay, C., Krelle, H., Idriss, O., Tallack, C. and Kelly, E. (2021) *Our ageing population: how ageing affects health and care need in England*, The Health Foundation [Online] Available from: https://doi.org/10.37829/HF-2021-RC16 [Accessed August 2023].

Sarter, E.K. and Cookingham Bailey, E. (2023) *Understanding public services: a contemporary introduction*, Policy Press.

Segall, M. (2018) 'We should scrap the internal market', article response, *BMJ*, 361: k2791 [Online] Available from www.bmj.com/content/361/bmj.k2791/rr [Accessed January 2024].

Shah, A. and Kanaya, A.M. (2014) 'Diabetes and associated complications in the South Asian population', *Current Cardiology Reports*, 16(5): 476. doi: 10.1007/s11886-014-0476-5

Social Care Institute for Excellence (2022) 'Co-production: what it is and how to do it' [Online] Available from: www.scie.org.uk/co-production/what-how/ [Accessed August 2023].

Stow, D., Hanratty, B. and Matthews, F.E. (2022) 'The relationship between deprivation and frailty trajectories over 1 year and at the end of life: a case-control study', *Journal of Public Health*, 44(4): 844–850.

Thaler, R.H. and Sunstein, C.R. (2008) *Nudge: improving decisions about health, wealth, and happiness*, Yale University Press.

UK Health Security Agency (2023) *Adverse Weather and Health Plan* [Online] Available from: https://assets.publishing.service. gov.uk/government/uploads/system/uploads/attachment_data/ file/1171545/Adverse-weather-health-plan-2023.pdf [Accessed August 2023].

West Suffolk Council (2022) 'Suffolk launches £150,000 match funder scheme for community action on the climate emergency', 7 July [Online] Available from: www.westsuffolk.gov.uk/news/ [Accessed August 2023].

Whitehead, M. (1991) 'The concepts and principles of equity and health', *Health Promotion International*, 6(3): 217–228.

Williams, E., Buck, D., Babalola, G. and Maguire, D. (2022) 'What are health inequalities?' *The King's Fund* [Online] Available from: www.kingsfund.org.uk/publications/what-are-health-inequalities [Accessed July 2023].

Index

References to figures appear in *italic* type; those in **bold** type refer to tables.